Healing Crystals and Gemstones for Beginners

Merge Chakras and Crystals Healing for More Power

FREDDIE SPENCER

Copyright © 2021 FREDDIE SPENCER

All rights reserved.

ISBN-13: 979-8-5090-3696-5

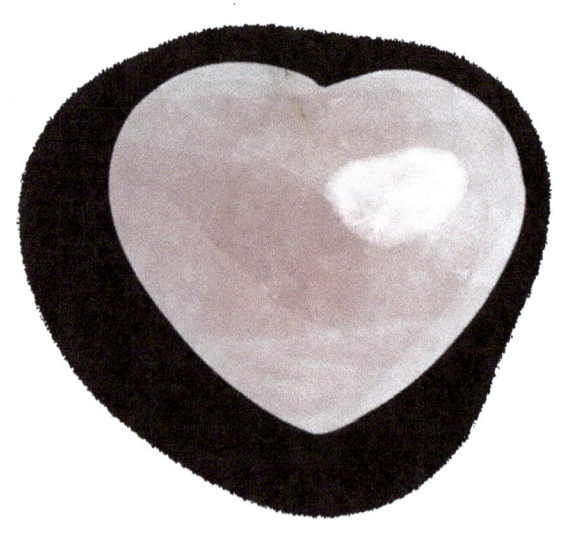

CONTENTS

INTRODUCTION

CHAPTER ONE

OVERVIEW ON CRYSTAL THERAPY

CHAPTER TWO

VISUALIZATION

CHAPTER THREE

CHOOSING YOUR CRYSTALS

CHAPTER FOUR

PROGRAMMING & CHARGE CRYSTALS

CHAPTER FIVE

HOW TO USE CRYSTALS FOR HEALING.

Crystals and Gemstones Alphabetical Index

CHAPTER SIX

CRYSTAL HEALING TIPS AND TECHNIQUES

4

INTRODUCTION

Crystal healing works due to the crystals' vibrational and enthusiastic levels. It repairs faults, regions, and tendencies within our vibrational energy fields.

You don't need to do anything extra to apply crystal healing; it's simply a piece of art. But you must be aware of what you are getting yourself into before you begin. Crystal therapy entails returning a person's energy to a more pleasant and changed state within their body to assist with a problem or change.

Crystal healing is a type of alternative medicine in which crystals and stones are used to treat illnesses and keep people from getting sick. This method acts as a therapeutic pathway, letting good, healing energy flow into the body while bad, infection-causing energy flows out.

In any case, healing crystals are still popular in wellness spas and New Age wellness centers, and they are sometimes used in back-rubbing and Reiki, which are similar practices. The use of crystals in such circumstances will aid in the induction of unwinding.

Crystal healers acknowledge that crystals and gemstones have characteristics that aid in recovery. The history of this instruction dates back at least 6,000 years, to the time of the ancient Sumerians of Mesopotamia. It is also said that the ancient Egyptians used gems like lapis lazuli, carnelian, and turquoise to keep disease and bad energy away.

Modern crystal healing is based on traditional ideas from Asian cultures, especially the Chinese idea of life-energy (chi or QI) and the Hindu or Buddhist idea of chakras, which are vortices of life-energy that connect the body's physical and spiritual parts.

Different characteristics are assigned to stones in crystal healing. However, healers have different ideas about which stones have particular characteristics. For example, amethyst is good for your digestive system, green aventurine is good for your heart, and yellow topaz helps you think more clearly. The seven chakras that focus on the body are associated with red to violet tones.

During a therapy session, a crystal healer may place various stones or crystals on your body that are aligned with specific chakra foci, often in the areas above the head, on the forehead, on the neck, on the chest, on the stomach, on the gut, and in the genital region. The stones are used, and where they are put may depend on how the patient is feeling. The healer's information comes from the chakra theory of illness and energy imbalance, which is a way of thinking that Western medical professionals often say is okay.

In crystal therapy, crystals and gemstones are also worn on the body or put under pillows to prevent infections, get rid of bad energy, or keep positive energy going.

Is crystal healing safe?

Many parents use Baltic gold neck bands to help their babies and young children feel less pain when they are getting their first teeth. This is similar to how different crystal stones are used to treat different illnesses. The reason for that is that the warmth of the child's skin releases a pain-relieving chemical (succinic acid) from the golden neckband, which is then absorbed into the bloodstream through the skin. The other is that the gold stimulates the thyroid to make the child drool more and reduces irritation in the ears, throat, stomach, and respiratory system.

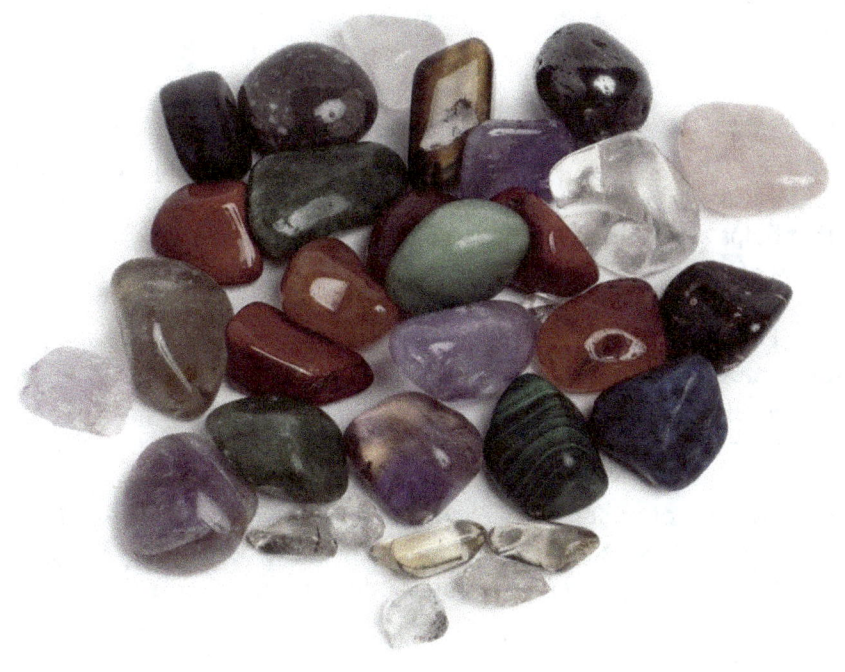

CHAPTER ONE

OVERVIEW ON CRYSTAL THERAPY

The crystal treatment is a treatment used to fix different infections, like agony and stress. The high-speed way of life and long working hours have brought forth disorders like pressure, tension, and body torment. This is a viable method that helps a great deal with unwinding. This treatment has been used since the days of yore.

In the crystal treatment, stones and crystals are widely used. It is widely accepted that these crystals aid in the healing of the body. A portion of the stones and crystals have a healing nature. These stones and crystals are put on the decisive parts to restore impact.

There are many kinds of crystals, and each one has its own healing power for the whole person. They spread good energy and help the body and brain get rid of bad energy, which is good for the body and the spirit.

Crystals are sold as old medicines that use ideas from Hinduism and Buddhism to explain how they work. This healing treatment is essentially pseudoscience. It is widely used to create an unwinding impact. These crystals, when applied to the skin, have an alleviating effect. The science behind this recovery treatment is that it invigorates the skin cells. At that point, this finally leads to the release of the chemicals and compounds that help you relax.

Everyone agrees that the unstoppable force of life has a cure for every disease. Different naturally occurring substances contain specific healing properties. People use these crystals to help the body get better and feel more alive.

The functioning standard of crystal treatment is straightforward. In this, the stones and crystals are given to the space of the body that is influenced by the torment. These work on the energy networks of the body. The crystals are used to eliminate antagonistic and hostile energy; this last outcome has a restoring impact on the body.

Different specialists are offering crystal treatment. No matter what, the fact that this treatment is so widely used shows that it works. This treatment has given a medical advantage to many individuals.

You can use the crystal treatment to get excellent help from the agony. The stones and crystals are set on the various pieces of the body, having been affected by the agony. This treatment is also effective at providing relaxation. The warmed structure's crystals and stones are placed on the head to provide relaxation. The secret recovering force helps eliminate the pressure and stress. This, in the end, has an alleviating impact on the psyche. The most ancient societies, like the Egyptians, Mayans, and Sumerians, knew about the supernatural powers of crystals and used them to decorate their bodies and buildings.

What Is the Process of Crystal Healing?

Over the last few hundred years, investigations into the structure of particles have revealed that everything in our universe is made up of energy. Even the most important things, like a household item or the hair on your head, are just vibrations of energy at the deepest levels. Even though it might not look like it, both recovering crystals and the cells in your body have energy.

Researchers have effectively sorted out some ways to use the energy intrinsic in crystals for a wide range of things, like keeping time using the tiny quartz crystals in your watch or making the electronic segments for your PC and cell phone. If you understand it, the fiery properties of crystal healing and stones are widely used in our cutting-edge innovation.

We even use crystals in our drugs. Numerous drugs are made by crushing minerals that form the structure of healing crystals. Even though our way of life has a few applications for the enthusiastic properties of crystals, we have failed to normalize their use in fiery healing.

Healing stones and crystals use energy in the same way that magnets do to attract or repel. When you place certain crystals over specific pieces of your body, your energy changes, vibrates, beats, and moves as per the properties and fiery mark of the crystal.

What Kind of Healing Can Crystals Provide?

You can use crystals to recover from everything, from headaches to nervousness. Healing crystals can also help you meditate faster, align your seven chakras, and even put you to sleep in the right circumstances. There's no restriction to the kinds or levels of healing you can get from the right crystal or stone in the right application.

If you want to heal a part of your mind, body, or soul, healing crystals can change your energy and get rid of awkwardness in three important ways:

Clearing: Crystals can retain and eliminate particular energy sources from your body. A recovering crystal can absorb negative energy from your body in the same way that a magnet can.

Stimulating: Healing crystals and stones can also send energy into your body, mind, or soul by setting off thunderous frequencies. This is like how power works by directing and moving energy into an item. A crystal can bridle energy from the quantum field and send it into your energy field. Try not to stress; in contrast to power, this crystal healing energy is effortless and not dangerous.

Adjusting: Our reality is exceptionally balanced. Take a gander at the leaves on trees or even your body. The energy of our planet, for example, changes things. Your point may be skewed here and there, and out of balance, healing crystals can use the properties mentioned above—drawing in and repelling—to adjust spaces of energetic disharmony.

Approaches to Use Healing Crystals

There are tons of different kinds of healing stones and crystals on the planet. There is an extraordinary measure of undiscovered healing power simply sitting out there, hanging tight for you! Nonetheless, before we plunge into sorting out what kind of crystal is ideal for your use, how about we go over some of the various ways you can use crystals to heal yourself?

Wear recovery crystals. Wearing particular crystals for healing can help you maintain a balanced energy field throughout the day because crystals and stones absorb, repel, and transmit energy. Think of the crystals you wear as nutrients. You eat the nutrient, and it supports your body for the whole day. Putting on your crystal adornments in the first part of the day or placing specific stones in your pocket resembles taking your everyday nutrients to an energetic level.

Spot recovering crystals on a particular piece of the body. Anyone who has heard of crystal healing has probably heard of this type of healing, which involves laying stones on the body. If you're searching for an immediate, explicit application, setting crystals on that piece of your body is a fantastic method to get to their healing properties. For instance, when you're injured, you apply a soothing balm to the injury. On the off chance that you have a migraine, you may put an unobtrusively placed quartz crystal on the spot of your torment.

Healing with stones and crystals is frequently a long process, so we should try to keep them, and they will contain a great deal of data about our experiences. Indeed, a quartz crystal can hold as much information as more than 22,000 iPhones, and that data doesn't get less important over time. By sitting with crystals and calming your mind while you think, you can often have amazing, life-changing experiences just by grabbing a fiery piece of history like that during the cycle.

Make use of a healing crystal lattice. When using a crystal network, you place particular crystal and stone types in a particular configuration. These patterns are designed to attract and transform energy. It may take some time to become proficient with all the different types of frameworks, but using a crystal lattice is an age-old therapeutic technique. However, many people find it terrific because it is an amazingly fantastic practice.

Rest close to them. Our psyches assume control when we are dozing, and it's an incredible chance to mend and learn at a speedy pace. By letting your crystals reline while you sleep, you can get rid of any fears or doubts that your rational brain might be showing. Take a try at putting crystals under your pad or on your bedside table and perceive what they mean for your fantasies and how you feel when you get up toward the beginning of the day.

Move them around the body. Crystals don't have to stand by to work adequately. In some cases, it's wiser to move stones and crystals all around your body to get the most healing impact from them. Try using a recovering crystal wand to get rid of bad energy fields all over your body, from your head to your toes. When practicing crystal healing, keep in mind that your energy field extends about three feet around you. Take this opportunity to address your entire quality.

Spot them in your home or vehicle. In the same way, you can use healing gemstones and crystals to help you reach a goal or do something you want to do. For instance, you can put defensive crystals in your car to hinder negative energy from mishaps or break-ins by setting that expectation into the crystal and then leaving it in those spots. You can use them similarly in your home or put the energy into a room. Crystals like rose quartz can also bring healing or loving energy into your room or near your tub.

Purifying and Aligning Your Crystals

Due to the fact that healing crystals absorb, attract, and repel specific types of energy, it is crucial to keep your crystals clean. If you use crystals to absorb negative energy, you must get rid of it before using them again. Consider this similar to using a wipe to absorb dirty water. If you want to continue using the wipe, you'll need to squeeze out the dirty, grimy water and clean it so the next dish you wash doesn't get dirty as well.

When you purchase healing crystals or stones in a store or online, they have retained and repelled the energy of every person who has touched them. Before you use them yourself, you'll need to purify their energy and adjust it to yours.

Doing this is essential. You can submerge your crystals in filtered water, saltwater, or holy water. However, do not submerge selenite or gold, as they will break apart. Similarly, crystals can be purified by smirching (using white sage, dried spices, or incense smoke). A few groups even give their regenerating crystals a "moon shower" by exposing them to the full moon's light in the evening.

After you've cleaned your healing stones and crystals, adjust them to your energy by holding them in the palm of your hand, closing your eyes, telling them what you want them to do for you, and thanking them for the healing they will give you.

At long last, clean your crystals after each use. This implies crystals you wear each day ought to be cleaned before you wear them the following day, and crystals used for a healing meeting ought to be speedily cleaned after every meeting.

Choosing Which Type of Crystal To Use

A crystal healing guide is a great way to figure out what crystals to use for different problems and situations. We've included one underneath to kick you off. In any case, your instinct will consistently be your best guide. You can ask the crystal or stone how they need to be used, ponder with it, use a pendulum, or go with your first sense.

Simply don't think so hard. Your rational brain doesn't generally know the appropriate response, yet your psyche does. Use your instinct and impulse, and you'll normally settle on the ideal decision.

White/Clear: Clearing

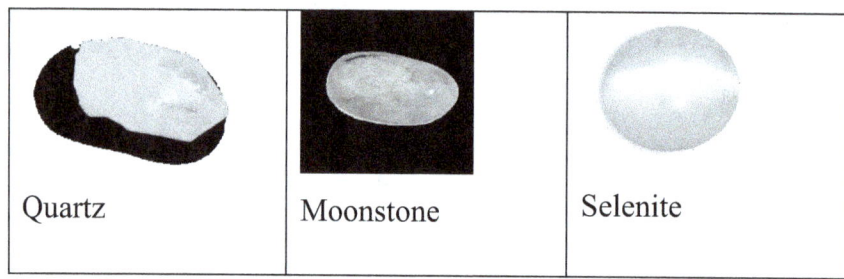

Models: Quartz, Moonstone, Selenite

Uses: White and clear recovering crystals are permeable. They are ideal for learning and purifying any sort of energy. Numerous people utilize clear quartz in their meditation practices because it clears and calms the mind. Make sure to clean your quartz often because it does retain its level.

Earthy colored: Allowing

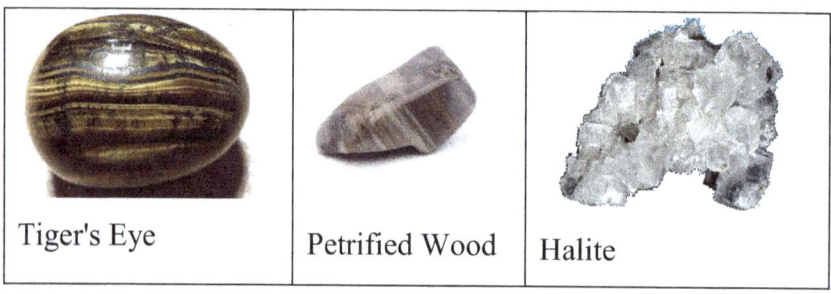

Models: Tiger's Eye, Petrified Wood, Halite

Uses: Brown crystal healing and stones are very established. When you consider earthy-colored crystals, think about a soil path in the mystery woods. This path shows you the way and ensures your safety on your excursion. That is what earthy colored stones do—control, confirm, and make room. Use them when you're attempting to make room in your life for something like a new position or relationship.

Red: Energizing

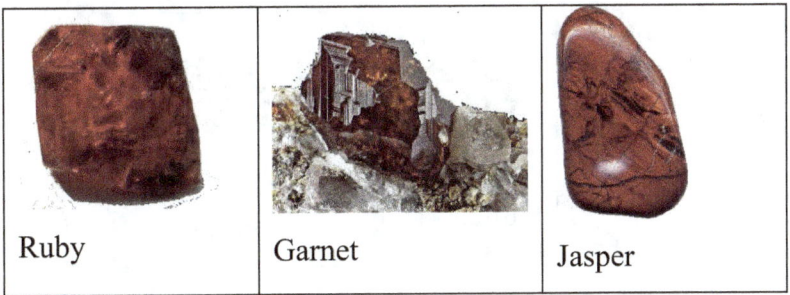

Models: Ruby, Garnet, Jasper

Uses: Red crystals have a ton of energy. You can help yourself remember this by thinking about your response to a red stop sign, a red traffic signal, or a red admonition signal. Red summons abrupt floods of energy, so on the off chance that you need a quick shot in the arm, you can heft around a red stone as a substitute for something unfortunate like a charged refreshment.

Orange: Releasing

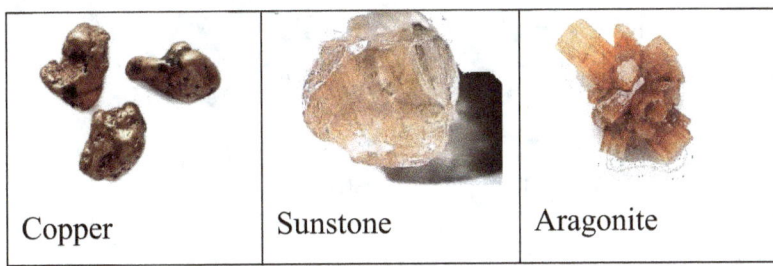

Models: Copper, Sunstone, Aragonite

Uses: You know how when you are truly incapacitated and walk outside and immediately feel much better? That is because orange have both a calming and stimulating tone. Orange healing stones get rid of bad energy and clear the way for more positive energy to flow. Use them when you're feeling sad or stalling.

Yellow: Aligning

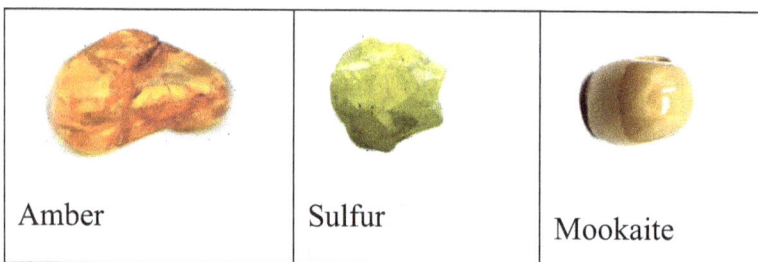

Models: Amber, Sulfur, Mookaite

Uses: Yellow crystal stones are incredible for revamping energy designs. These crystals are great when you want to teach someone a new habit or break a bad one. Consider yellow stones to be a material of exceptional quality. They don't simply scrub energy; they revamp it.

Green: Balancing

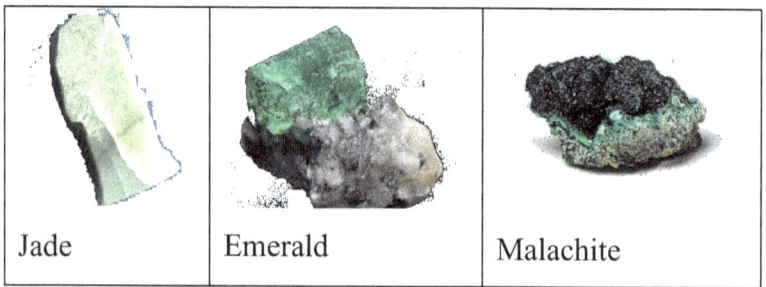

Models: Jade, Emerald, Malachite

Uses: Green crystal stones are frequently used for actual recovery, given their adjusting properties. Regularly, our illnesses involve a lot of things. For example, stomach-related issues are frequently caused by a large number of corrosive bacteria or unfortunate microorganisms. While we need these things to endure, many of them make us debilitated. Green healing stones do not eliminate negative energy; rather, they steer the results in the right direction by redirecting and adjusting our energy flows.

Blue: Communicating

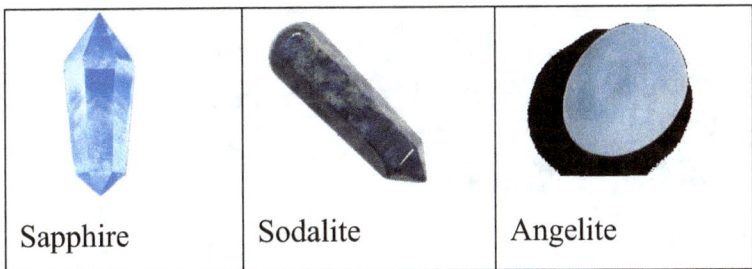

Models: Sapphire, Sodalite, Angelite

Uses: Like the blue throat chakra, blue recovering crystals are about receptiveness and correspondence. Use blue crystals for healing if you are having trouble finding your facts or if you need the truth to be revealed about something.

Indigo: Calming

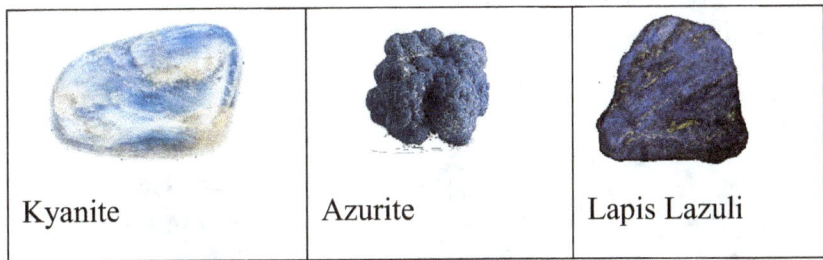

Models: Kyanite, Azurite, Lapis Lazuli

Occasionally use: When life becomes truly chaotic, you simply need to unwind and relax. Next time you need to get yourself a quiet spa experience, use the mitigating force of dim blue or indigo healing crystal stones to relax restless, delicate energy.

Violet: Uplifting

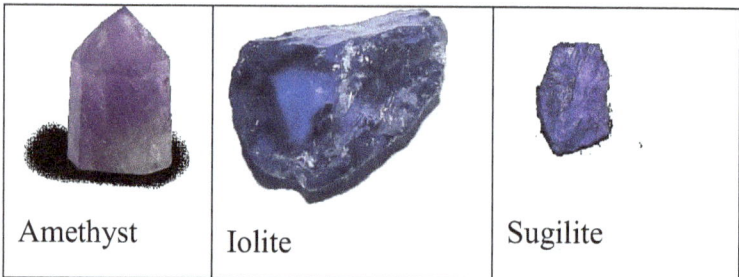

Models: Amethyst, Iolite, Sugilite

Violet is possibly the most remarkable tone due to its high recurrence and frequency of vibration. It is at the highest point of our shading range, joining both the warm and cool closures of the multitude of tones we can see. Along these lines, anything violet associates you with a higher plane of presence. There is no exemption to the beauty of violet healing crystals. You should be elevated; you need to incite a profound encounter or approach higher forces to manage you.

Dark: Protecting

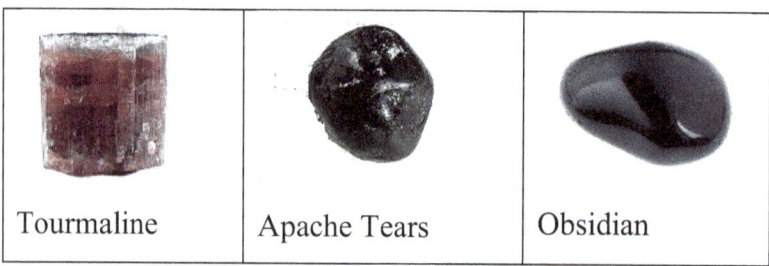

Models: Tourmaline, Apache Tears, Obsidian

Uses: Black healing crystals divert everything. They are solid and rigid, so they make unique ensuring crystals. On the off chance that you need to repel any sort of energy, use dark stones to drive those negative energies away from you.

Pink: Loving

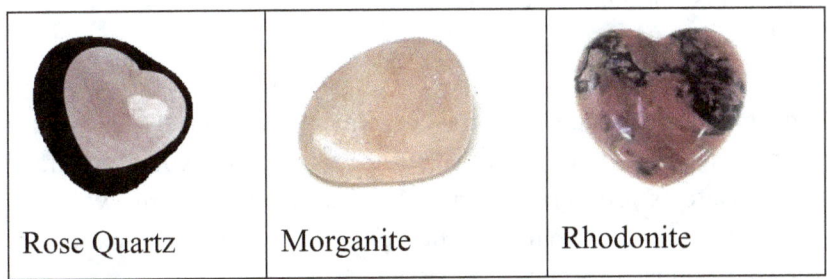

| Rose Quartz | Morganite | Rhodonite |

Models: Rose Quartz, Morganite, Rhodonite

Uses: Pink makes us consider sentiment, and that is because the shading pink is a mix of enthusiastic red and explaining white. However, you don't need to use pink healing crystals only for the sentiment. They vibrate with a humane, cherishing energy, so use them for anything that needs a smidgen of pleasantness. They are great for avoiding anger, getting people to feel something, or just making you feel love.

Various kinds of healing crystals

Clear quartz

This white crystal is viewed as an "ace healer." It's said to enhance energy by engrossing, putting away, delivering, and directing it. It's additionally said to help fixation and memory. In fact, it is believed that transparent crystals can assist in balancing the immune system and the entire body. This stone is frequently combined with others, such as rose quartz, in order to enhance and strengthen their properties.

Rose quartz

Similarly, as the tone may suggest, this pink stone is about adoration. It's said that it will help rebuild trust and agreement in all of their relationships while strengthening the ones close to them. It is also said to provide comfort and peace during times of sadness.

Rose quartz also promotes self-love, self-respect, self-confidence, and self-worth, which is something we could all use these days.

Jasper

This lustrous crystal is regarded as the "preeminent nurturer." It engages the soul, supporting you through times of stress by preparing you to eventually "appear." It protects you from negative energies and keeps them away. It also gives you courage, quick thinking, and confidence. These are extra-useful qualities while handling significant issues, which is by and large what this stone might be helpful for.

Obsidian

A strongly defensive stone, obsidian helps structure a safeguard against physical and enthusiastic pessimism. It additionally helps dispose of energetic blockage and advance the characteristics of solidarity, clarity, and empathy to help track down your actual ability to be self-aware. It might help with digestion and detoxification, and it might also make your body feel better and cause less pain.

Citrine

Bring happiness, miracles, and eagerness to all aspects of your existence with citrine. It's said to help you discharge negative characteristics from your life, like dread, and empower positive thinking, warmth, inspiration, and transparency. It also improves careful abilities such as imagination and focus.

Turquoise

This blue crystal has powers that help recuperate the whole self. As a rule, it's viewed as a rabbit's foot that can help balance your feelings while tracking down your metaphysical foundations. Regarding the body, it's said to benefit the respiratory, skeletal, and invulnerable frameworks.

Tiger's eye

If you need help with force or inspiration, this brilliant stone could be for you. It aids in the release of your psyche and collection of dread, uneasiness, and self-doubt. This can be helpful for vocation desires or even matters of the heart. Tiger's eye is also intended to help you achieve harmony and balance in order to make more conscious decisions.

Amethyst

This purple stone is extraordinarily defensive, healing, and purifying. It is guaranteed to assist in clearing the mind of negative thoughts and delivering serenity, candor, and profound insight. Additionally, it promotes connectivity. Another asserted benefit of this stone, as far as anyone knows, is that it aids in the alleviation of sleeping disorders and the acquisition of dreams. Indeed, it helps chemical creation, scrubs blood, and assuages agony and stress.

Moonstone

Known for "fresh starts," moonstone is said to energize internal development and strength. When starting something new, this stone is suspected to mitigate those uncomfortable sensations of stress and precariousness, so you're ready to push ahead effectively. It is said again to improve positive thinking, instinct, and motivation while bringing success and good luck.

Bloodstone

This incredible healing stone lives up to its name. Bloodstone is said to help clean the blood by getting rid of bad natural energies and making the blood flow better. Talking carefully makes you more generous, creative, and optimistic, and it also helps you live in the moment. It additionally helps you free yourself of sensations of touchiness, forcefulness, and anxiety.

Sapphire

This blue stone is one of cunning and eminence. It's said it can pull in success, joy, and harmony while opening up the brain to acknowledge magnificence and instinct. In terms of physical health, this stone is used to treat eye problems, low cell counts, and blood disorders. It is also used to treat depression, anxiety, and trouble sleeping.

Ruby

A red champion, this stone restores essentials and energy levels. This can help improve things like exotic nature, sex, and insight. Likewise, it's to help bring mindfulness and the acknowledgment of truth to one's psyche. Rubies were used in ancient times to help eliminate poisons from the blood and, generally speaking, improve the circulatory framework.

Step-by-step instructions to choose your crystal

Firstly, identify what you feel you're missing before investigating what stones can give you. This will assist you with demonstrating what's happening inside yourself before relying upon outside sources.

From that point on, just let your instinct pick what's best for you. Regardless of whether a crystal grabs your attention or you feel an actual draw toward one, your internal psyche will help guide you to the crystal that is appropriate for you. When it's selected, you can make the association you need.

The most effective method to focus on your crystal

When you first bring your crystal home, you'll need to clean it to get rid of any dirt or grime it may have picked up. You can hold it under chilly, running water from a tap or wash it in a characteristic wellspring of water. In any case, be sure the water is calm, not warm or hot.

Add a little bit of ocean salt to clean it up, or eat sage to help it get rid of bad energies. Likewise, you can't forget about letting it dry in morning daylight or full moon light to let the light channel through.

It's not just about their actual consideration, however. For crystals to do something unique, you intellectually need to eliminate the negative energy or doubt you may have about their capacities. It's imperative to consider how they can help you.

Crystal frill

Crystals may be best known for their ability to heal, but if we're honest, they're also beautiful. So it's nothing unexpected; individuals make vast loads of extras out of them, similar to crystals or home beautification. Not only will the crystals look decent, but keeping great energy around never hurts anybody.

Supplication dots

Crystal petition dabs are worn against the heart to inspire a variety of positive emotions, regardless of anticipation, grit, or harmony. They're an incredible path for anybody to raise around the recovering forces of crystals.

Adornments

Adornments are another fantastic way to enhance a crystal's abilities. Likewise, it permits you to flaunt each stone's excellence.

Liners

These staggering liners are produced using veritable crystal stones from Brazil. The agate stone in this family matter will help advance equilibrium and congruity inside the home. These are ideal for individuals who need to bring great energies into their dwelling place.

Sex toys

These crystal sex toys work by combining their energies with your sexual energy to give you pure sexual pleasure. They're fantastic tools for people who have been in a sexual trench to help them open up.

Lines

In all honesty, you can even check out crystal-made hand pipes. They're smooth, simple to use, and solid. This makes them an extraordinary present for any individual who uses clinical weed to deal with a medical issue.

Water bottles

Stylish water bottles are currently just about as popular as crystals, so it's not surprising that the two have been combined. On the lower part of these beautiful glass bottles sits a "diamond unit." It's said to advance everything from health and excellence to adjustment. This is the ideal assistant to bring to your next yoga practice.

A receptive outlook is vital to acquiring these delightful stones' positive characteristics. There's nothing wrong with trying crystals, whether you're looking for general energy or specific healing powers. Who knows, you may be enjoyably astounded.

Think about Using Crystal Therapy to Survive the Daily Grind

Life can be very distressing now and again. Going to work every day and taking care of different obligations can drain your energy. You can feel baffled with day-by-day frustrations that can go from an illness to proficiency issues to love issues and even the critical factors of a coming test or an advancement. If you need to take a healing break from these things, you can use crystal therapy. You can use it to help heal an illness, change your energy, protect yourself from bad energy, and, surprisingly, find love in this world. Here are some significant points about which you should think about crystal treatment.

The Basics of Crystal Therapy

The belief in crystal treatment is based on the conviction that specific crystals and appeal stones have a significant impact on the balancing of energies within us. It is possible that we as a whole have some sort of vibrational energy framework, and the use of these energy stones and crystals can do a lot to protect this framework. So, these beautiful stones hold magical or healing powers and can be used without the help of a crystal expert. The effectiveness of this sort of treatment would be put together not just concerning the capacity to draw a crystal's forces out but also in addition to the stone's compound, its sort, tone, nuclear construction, and its actual structure. This means that a particular crystal can have special powers that can be used to meet specific needs. In any case, as a rule, there is the possibility that a solitary charm stone contains one sort of healing power as well as a few.

If you want to use crystal therapy for healing, here is a guide to the different crystals and stones and how they work.

1. Chakra Balancers

There are certain crystals that can help you adjust your energy. This is a decent spot to begin on the off chance that you don't know which center space you would need. To have a generally adjusted nature at that point, you can use jade, serpentine, and fulgurite as your chakra adjusting stones.

2. Love Crystals

Assuming you need to find support in the space of affection, you can use love crystals. The most famous ones are rose quartz, apatite, and cobalt calcite. These appeal stones give off warm and gentle energies, which makes them great for attracting love or helping you understand what other people are going through.

3. Invigorating Charm Stones

If you are low on energy, you can use unique necklaces, rings, or some other crystal piece with opal or topaz stones as a feature of your crystal therapy. These appealing stones can help you when you are debilitated and exhausted. Simply make sure to get them far from your bedside so you can have a decent night's rest.

4. Memory Keepers

Some stones help the mind remember things, which is why they are also called "crystal record managers." A few models incorporate rubies, garnets, and carnelians. They can be precious when you are planning for tests.

5. Defensive and Shielding Crystals

Jewels, yellow jasper, and fluorite are the best defensive appeal stones. They work best when worn as an accessory or kept in a suitcase or pocket. These crystals work by absorbing the negative energies around you, so it's also important to know how to clean them from time to time.

predominantly intends to adjust the energy inside you. Crystal treatment, which is mostly about adjusting your energy, requires that you use the crystals we've already talked about. Crystal therapy is also thought to heal and relax the body and mind, as well as strengthen the body's immune system.

ADVANTAGE OF CRYSTAL THERAPY

Crystal treatment has been used for quite a long time to help treat the body comprehensively for different afflictions, and the use of these precious minerals traces back to Egyptian occasions when they were supposed to be used to cleanse 'detestable spirits.'

Crystal therapy is based on the idea that certain stones, like amethyst, rose quartz, and jade, can communicate with the body's energy flow and help to realign the energy channels that are getting in the way of the body's normal flow and help it heal itself. Certain crystals with certain stones can help with mental illnesses like anxiety, depression, and lack of sleep, as well as physical illnesses like stomach problems.

Crystal therapy can be just as important as wearing valuable stones and minerals as bracelets and necklaces, putting crystals in the room where you work and sleep, or being treated by a crystal specialist who knows which stones can try to energize the seven chakras, or "energy centers," around the body.

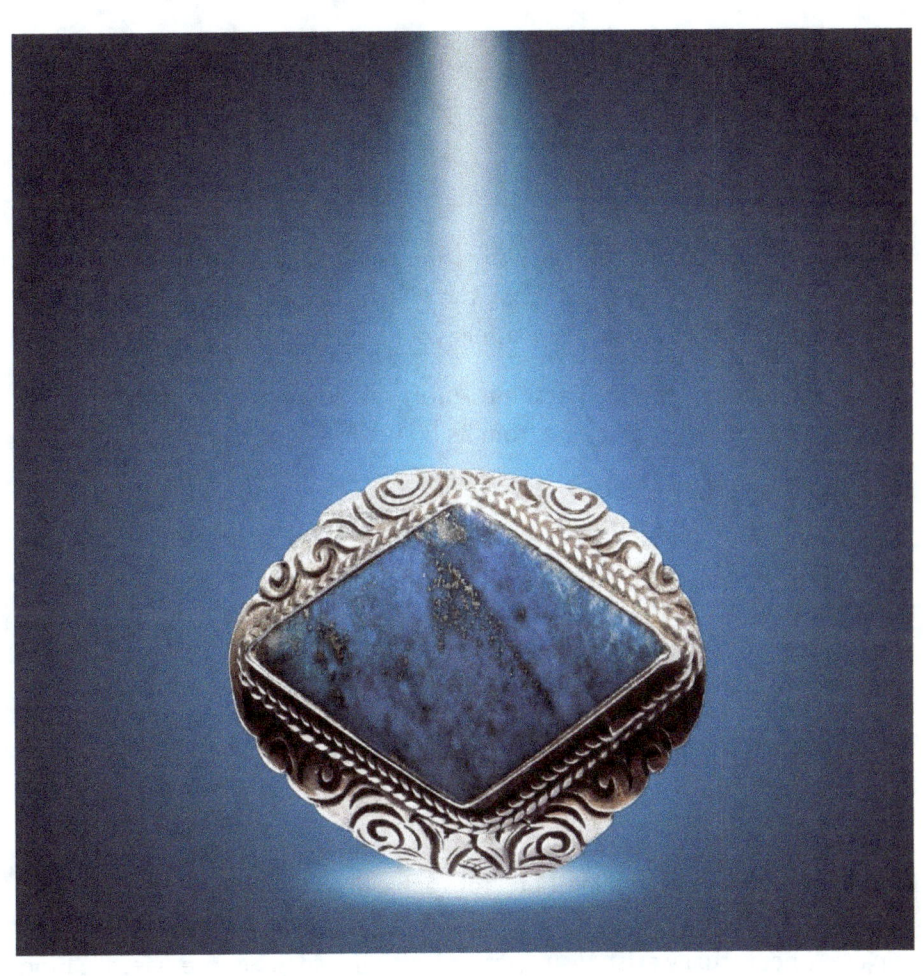

CHAPTER TWO

VISUALIZATION

Visualization expects you to need something, see it, and put stock in it. After a while, as you work toward your goal, the interaction and energy you put into perception will begin to positively affect your life.

While visualization sets aside some effort to dominate, there are a few different ways to begin profiting from its influences right away.

Envision yourself by opening the fridge. Imagine yourself taking out a lemon. Hold the lemon in your palms. Feel the surface of its waxy, yellow strip and its perfection, and feel the yellow ribbon finishing at a point. Marginally press the lemon in your palm and feel the presence of a new squeeze inside. Take a sharp blade and cut the lemon into two parts. Lemon scent atoms are newly delivered to your nose. Smell the lemon scent. Presently, nibble the lemon.

On the off chance that your mouth has salivated at this point, you just had an incredible visualization experience. You haven't chomped into the lemon, yet your mouth has actually salivated. That is the force of visualization.

Visualization is a great method for achieving goals in everyday life. Visualization implies completing something as a top priority. However, that thing may not actually exist. Visualization isn't a magic thing. The "visualization of progress" is a procedure to be performed based on discoveries made by specialists after research. Notably, competitors and athletes are instructed to rehearse perception strategies for top execution.

Specialists now ground it in the field, where every creation you see around you began as a thought. Everything, like the structures, the vehicles, the streets, the furnishings, the pen, the paper, and the PC, was first imagined in somebody's mind for quite a while. Each creation, including you and me, has its birthplace as a top priority. God first pictured us quite a while ago and made us in His image.

If you want to succeed at something, wouldn't it make sense to first picture yourself succeeding? Surely it is. Allow me to show you how.

I have been rehearsing this perception strategy in my life for a long time. When I was a different legal counselor, I frequently imagined myself standing confidently in front of judges, on my feet, and effectively arguing my client's case.

Visualization strategies have helped me enormously in my prosperity as an attorney. I keep on rehearsing this visualization procedure even at this point. With my eyes shut and keeping in mind that hitting the sack, I in a real sense find to my eyes, the court in the entirety of its subtleties; the Honorable adjudicators sitting on the dais; I hear my case being called out by the Court Reader; me strolling surely and moving toward the Bar; and starting my contention discourse in a sure style; confronting the court inquiries readily and keeping up my balance all through and still, at the end of the day assaulted with troublesome inquiries; fulfilling the court and convincing them in my mind; the way of my elocution; the tone of discourse; my motions and so forth

You can apply this perception procedure to prevail in any part of your life. You can make better connections, like going out with the most beautiful girl and having a great relationship with your partner. Also, you might have the chance to get better at things like public speaking and driving a car. You can even figure out how to be more sure and decisive using perception strategies, like moving toward the manager for a raise or advancement or denying something you would prefer not to do. You can also practice perception to make progress in any area of your life.

- Identify the part of your life which you need to prevail.

- Practice visualization consistently while heading to sleep and each day on arousing.

- Close your eyes and make mental pictures during visualization.

- Let your psychological pictures be in as much detail as expected.

- Have the visualization experience through your own eyes. This implies that you need to imagine as though you're in reality. You ought not to glance at yourself from a third individual's perspective.

- See yourself dominant in your undertaking during your visualization cycle.

- During perception experience, blend your feelings in with the experience.

Accept, without reservation, that what you envision will emerge as a general rule. Remember that your visualization experience isn't just for fun. You are creating and submitting a request to the universe for your craving goal.

To accomplish the best outcomes, disguise the envisioned insight. Allow it to turn into a piece of your being.

Understanding the role of the brain in motivation and behavior may be the most basic idea for real health success. On the off chance that you battle with changing propensities and practices or assume you can't be persuaded, even the best preparation and nourishment program is useless.

An interesting reality about your non-cognizant brain is that it's deductive. It is completely equipped for working in reverse, from the finish to the methods. You don't have to have a plan or the "know-how" to reach a goal when you first set it. If you "program" just the result (the ideal) into your "psychological PC," your inner mind will take over and help you find the necessary information, ways, and actions to reach your ideal end.

Numerous individuals know about confirmations and objective-setting strategies to offer directions to your psyche. Yet, maybe a definitive method to take advantage of the great forces of your psyche is to use the strategy called perception. In one way, persistence and perception are the same, because when you say or think a confirmation first, it sets off a mental picture because the human brain "thinks" in pictures.

You can use visualization to program objectives into your subconscious mind. It's basic: You close your eyes and visualize and film how you want things to turn out. For instance, you can envision your body, in as striking a point of interest as could be expected, precisely how you need it to look. When you repeat mental pictures to yourself over and over, your subconscious takes them as orders to be carried out. This helps you change habits, behaviors, and performance.

Advantages

Increment inspiration

For persuasive visualization to work, you have to picture yourself reaching your ultimate goal and feeling the emotions that come with it. Invigorate every one of your faculties and immerse yourself in a psychological picture so that a lot of it comes across as genuine to you. By acclimating yourself to sensations of accomplishment, you increase your inspiration to arrive at your ultimate objective and accept that achievement is more conceivable and practical.

Characterize what you need

Figure out how to remove your consideration from what you don't need and zero in on what you wish to encounter. Visualization lets us get rid of all the negative feelings that come with pessimism and instead focus on doing things that will help us grow as individuals. When you've defined your goal, keep practicing perception on a regular basis. The more definite your perception, the closer your goal will appear to you.

Increment positive contemplations

For the day, we have a continuous inward discourse with ourselves. Be aware of your thoughts and choose them carefully. You should be a friend to yourself, not a dangerous enemy. By expanding positive contemplations today, you start to welcome positive results into your life. You will not begin to see changes the first day, but supporting them is like sowing a seed. Promptly, you will feel more joyful, and after some time, things will start to move in your life.

Upgrade execution

One sort of mental symbolism that builds our presentation is picturing yourself in high-pressure circumstances. You can create adapting procedures and better react to future tensions by mentally preparing for testing conditions. Jim Bauman, Ph.D., the counseling sports clinician for USA Swimming, says to name something near you that will remind you to keep a solid point of view when times get tough. For instance, the letter "P" on your PC can remind you to take a perspective that centers around your resources and not on the wrong considerations.

Diminish pressure

Perception is perhaps the ideal approach to get your brain in the groove again when you feel out of equilibrium. Listening to calm music and imagining your day can help you sort out your worries, get your mind ready for the day, and feel less stressed. Another way to relieve stress is to lie on your back and imagine all the tension in your body as warm magma gathering at the top of your head. This is my all-around favorite method. At that point, gradually expect it to pour down your ears, neck, shoulders, and whole body. You ought to feel a sensation move down your body as you expect the pressure to leave your head. I use this to nod off, and I have never remained conscious past my shoulders.

Imaginative visualization implies making a picture or a scene or envisioning something for yourself, with eyes open or shut. Then, that picture, scene, or creative thought is used to replace any pain or deal with any bad luck by adding good feelings. In any case, imaginative visualization isn't just about managing torment or misfortune. It additionally helps support confidence, improve temperaments, battling nervousness, and so on

Our minds can conjure up some truly fascinating scenarios. These things shouldn't be genuine or even bode well. Our psyche will envision it on the off chance that it is comprehensible. Innovative visualization is powerful because it can change how we think, feel, and act in social situations.

The cerebrum is equipped for making two kinds of pictures. Allow us to see them in detail:

1. Visual Imagery

This type of creative visualization is the place where a picture can be seen, voices can be heard, and now and again, you may even feel the impacts. Visual symbolism is used in the most inventive perception.

Ordinarily, when we envision a seashore or any type of water, we envision a lovely shore, the sound of the sea, and, if you are exceptionally imaginative, you can even feel the sand beneath your feet!

2. Non-Visual Imagery

This is when there is no image development in the brain. Yet, any remaining faculties together assist in envisioning. So, when a well-trained performer tunes his instruments or tries to remember a piece of music, non-visual symbols play a big role. He can hear the sound or feel the instrument's strings and judge if everything is in order or not.

Innovative perception firmly affects individuals. How we think, respond, carry on, and so forth can be adjusted with the assistance of creative visualization. Allow us to take a gander at the advantages of creative visualization.

Above all else, having a creative mind has benefits in every part of life. It is widely used in medicine and other circumstances where these sorts of innovative visualizations prove helpful.

- Therapeutic Benefits

If a person has different mental problems, he or she needs to be able to see things in new ways. If a person is experiencing anxiety, they are asked to imagine peaceful, quiet, and relieving scenes. The hints of the ocean are played, and they come slowly, envisioning a coastline. This assists them with quieting down without using any medicine.

When a person is going through real pain, they are told to think of easy and pleasant things while the other drug works. This is done because, when in torment, steady consideration regarding the agony exacerbates it.

• Forgetting Fear

Frequently, individuals suffer from sudden anxiety at the last possible moment. This is regular, yet it turns into an obstacle to their presentation. Be it in front of an audience, in a test lobby, or anyplace. To deal with such a circumstance, one can imagine post-triumphant scenes. This helps us get over our nerves and put forth a strong effort.

• Morale Booster

Now and then, our resolve goes down. We feel low and are not spurred enough to complete things. Through creative thinking, we can get our brains to picture all the beauty and rewards that are waiting for us at the end of the journey. This assists us with getting up and, at any rate, starting.

A similar perception likewise assists us with finishing assignments once we start them.

• Mood promoter

Most of the time, if we are getting more sure, gentle pressure and feeling more euphoria, our mood will be good as well. When we dream of every one of those things that fulfill us, we naturally set up the interaction of failing to remember our issues.

Phases of Creative Visualization

1. Picture Generation

Here the picture appears. We start envisioning and framing a psychological view once in a while from memory, from a dream, and some of the time from both.

2. Picture Maintenance

Here, we attempt to keep the picture alive. Our psyche is inclined to forget without any problem. As a result, this progression is linked to keeping the image alive long enough for us to consider it genuine.

3. Picture Inspection

Presently, our brain might be distracted. However, it has an incredible consideration for detail. So the next step is to look closely at the picture to make it look as real as possible. This includes contrasting the image with other mental images and our real encounters.

4. Picture Transformation

This is the last and most significant advance, making it genuine. The picture that was just essential for the psyche is now capable of being experienced by the brain and body. In the last step, the effects of the symbolism, such as easing, calming, reducing, and so on, are felt and enjoyed.

Creative visualization is considerably more troublesome than we give our minds credit for. It can regularly be a depleting experience, indeed, both inwardly and outwardly. As that may be, when we do it, we are frequently left with a feeling of profound quiet and tranquility when we accomplish imaginative visualization. Issues appear to settle themselves, and we are left inclination loose.

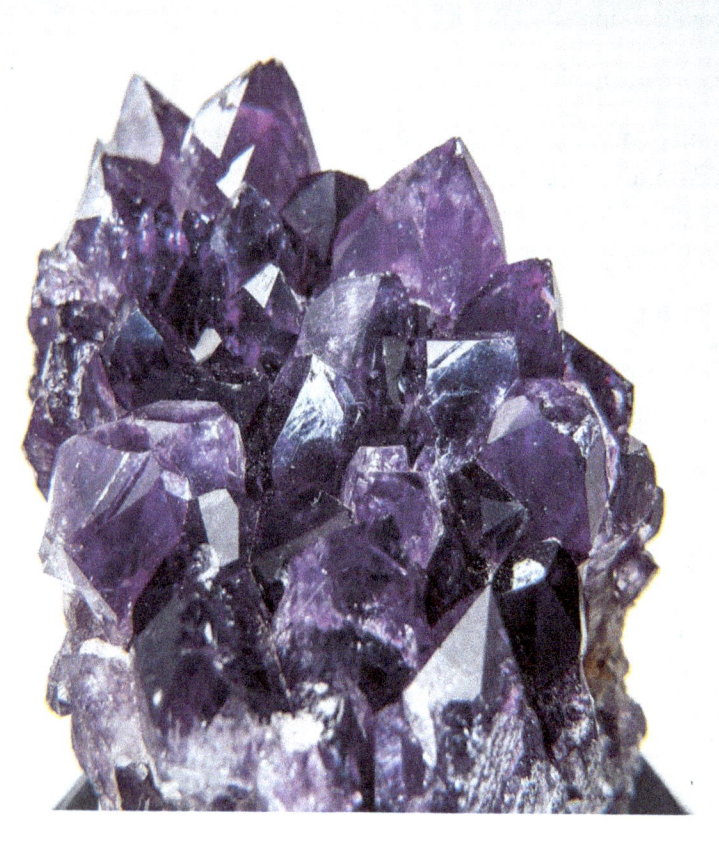

CHAPTER THREE

CHOOSING YOUR CRYSTALS

Make sure you have at least two of each basic color you'll be using when choosing crystals for your own use and beginning. This incorporates the colors red, orange, yellow, green, blue, purple, pink, white, clear, and dark. The colors of crystals correspond to our chakra centers and can also be compared to certain diseases. When working, it is a good idea to have a wide range of crystals and gemstones to choose from.

My undisputed top choices to keep available are Peridot, Hematite,

Red Jasper, Rose Quartz, Rhodonite, Carnelian, Topaz,

Golden, Tiger's Eye, Malachite, Bloodstone, Moss Agate,

Turquoise, Aquamarine, Lapis Lazuli, Amethyst, Fluorite,

Clear Quartz, Moonstone, Onyx, Black Tourmaline, and

Smoky Quartz.

There are numerous crystals and gemstones available, so avoid becoming overwhelmed and confused when deciding which ones are best for you or worried if you didn't get the right ones. The best manual for picking your crystals is to follow your instinct. If you listen to your instinct, it will never misguide you. Occasionally, it can be difficult to comprehend if you have not previously practiced following your "gut" instincts, but when working with crystals, it is important to listen to them.

When you first go out to select your new crystals, you should be optimistic and in a good mood. You would prefer not to attract negative fiery emotions, so put on some upbeat music in the vehicle and consider something that you appreciate while you are headed to the crystal shop.

When you arrive, proceed to begin glancing around to perceive what gets your attention first. Get the crystal and check whether it feels right to you. If it does, search for additional crystal healing units to add to your own. On the off chance that it doesn't, put it down and move to another!

The only correct response is the one that resonates within you! Simply keep in mind that your crystals will choose you regardless of how much you like them!

PURIFYING YOUR CRYSTALS

All crystals and crystal stones should be purified before use. You have no clue about where they have been, who has been getting them checked to see if they were a correct fit for their energy fields, or what sorts of energies are now connected to them. So the principal thing you need to do when you get them home is scrub them!

There are a couple of different approaches to scrubbing your new crystals. You can use smirching, water purging, Mother Earth's energy, sage tea purifying, sunlight-based energy, sound vibrations, reflecting the energy, and even sand purging if you decide.

To scrub your crystals with smirching, hold them within the smoke of your smear stick. Smearing with unadulterated wisdom or a wise blend turns out best for crystal purging. Pass them through the cloud of smoke multiple times back and forth.

Purifying your crystals with water and ocean salt is straightforward. For the more complex crystals, you can put them in a glass compartment of ocean salt water for at least 60 minutes. For the milder crystals, you can fog them liberally with a water splash to cover the crystals and have a lot of run-off.

Using Mother Earth's energy is an essential and fun, yet messy, way to purge your crystals. Wrap your crystal in cheesecloth and then in silk. Track down a unique spot in your yard where you can cover your new crystal. Create a hole 6 to 8 inches wide and 8 to 12 inches deep, then place your crystal inside. Cover it, and make sure to put a marker on it so you can uncover it! After 24 hours, locate your crystals and carefully remove any loose soil from them.

Sage tea purification is a fun and risk-free method for combining a variety of perspectives for an extraordinary crystal cleansing gathering. Take some new savvy, on the off chance you have it, and brew a pot of tea produced using the new wit. Permit this to cool, and then place your crystals in a glass bowl. Pour the sage-infused tea over the crystals and permit it to wash for the time being. This uses the strength of smirching and water energy to scrub them. Make sure to flush them toward the beginning of the day!

Sun-powered energy and water can be used for purifying crystals, too. You can do this by holding the crystals under running water briefly and then setting the crystals in the sun to dry. A few crystals may blur with the primary beams of the sun, so try not to leave them in direct sunlight for too long. It just requires a couple of moments for them to dry, so watch out for them!

The use of sound vibrations is another superb method to purge crystals with pure sound. A ringer or tuning fork can be used for this. Use your ringer or tuning fork to make its vibrational sound and spot the crystals as close as possible to the chime or tuning fork without intruding on the vibration.

Using mirror energy to scrub crystals and crystal stones is exceptionally simple. Place your crystal on top of a mirror, put it on your table or dresser, and permit the mirror to reflect back and out the energy that the crystals are now holding. Permit this to stay in the mirror for, in any event, 24 hours.

A sand technique can also be used on almost any kind of crystal or crystal stone. Cover your crystal in wet sand and leave it for at least 2 hours. Kindly note that the sand can eliminate a portion of the clean from the crystals, so just use this if all else fails.

When you use your crystals in healing sessions or for crystal gridding, you should regularly cleanse them. Each issue is unique and must be evaluated based on what the healing or gridding is attempting to accomplish with its mission. One important general rule is that you should always clean your crystals after each individual healing session. When working with gridding situations, these can shift from purging once per week to once a month. Crystals that are worn should be cleaned and then made new every so often, if necessary. Kindly follow the rules in this book for the best outcomes.

If you use crystal healing work regularly, whether for yourself or for other people, remember that the healing is done by the crystals. It is consistently a smart idea to send them home to Mother Earth for at least one month during a scheduled year when they are used frequently. I intend to cover them in Mother Earth in order to re-energize their vibrational healing. Ensure your stamps are where you hid them, and write in your schedule to remind you when to uncover them once more!

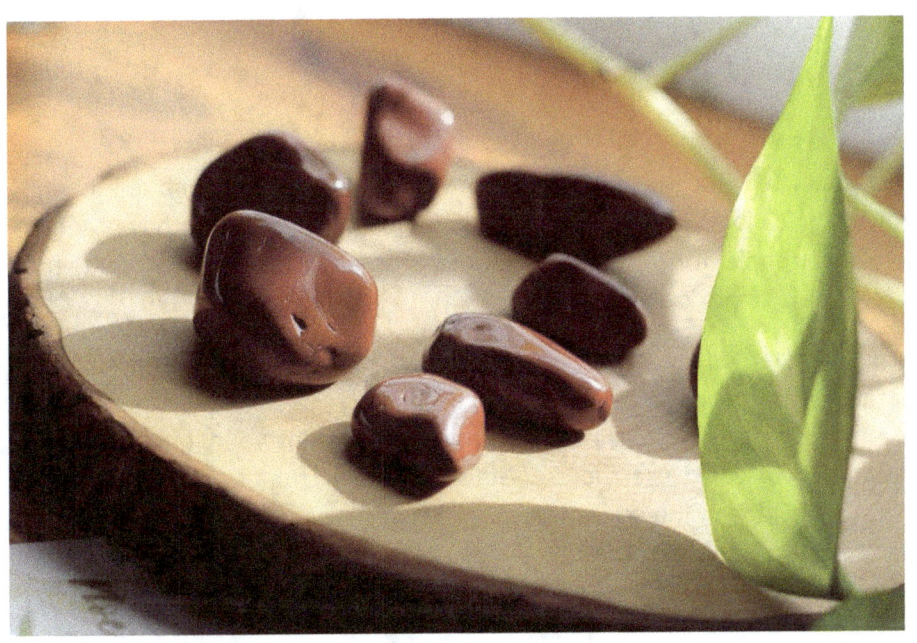

CHAPTER FOUR

PROGRAMMING & CHARGE CRYSTALS

Programming or charging crystals is a way to work with them and tell them, through their vibrations, what you want them to do while you have them. There are a couple of different ways you can program or charge them, yet their straightforwardness is awesome!

The passive method is probably the easiest way to teach a crystal or gemstone what to do. This is finished by just using a similar crystal for similar purposes. For instance, you wish to use a specific Amethyst during your contemplation meetings. You would use these crystals repeatedly for the same purpose. Doing this will teach the crystals to do what they are meant to do, which will help you on your journey to other worlds in the long run.

The Active Method requires slightly more focus and concentration, but can still be fun! This is done by focusing your thoughts, goals, attention, and heart on what you want to achieve while using this particular crystal or gemstone. Recall that your goal should be congruent with the crystals for everything to fall into place. For instance, you can't use the dynamic strategy to program an Amethyst to be used for establishing work. These two vibrational levels won't relate, and the programming won't "stick" with the crystal. You could, as the case may be, use the dynamic technique with an amethyst for issues like cerebral pain, instinct, sleep deprivation, and numerous other reasons. Establishing isn't a trait for working with an amethyst, so the vibrational levels won't coordinate.

You can likewise charge a crystal or gemstone with Reiki. This strengthens the connection between you and the crystal and enhances the crystal's normal capabilities. You should be receptive to, at any rate, a Reiki Level I to have the option to do this, or you can have somebody who is sensitive to Reiki charge the crystals for you. It is an essential and straightforward undertaking to perform. Take the crystal or crystal stone between the palms of your hands and start your Reiki stream. Then, request that the crystal be restored, and grant it access to this Reiki energy to assist its motivations with your direction.

Continue to channel your Reiki energy until the crystal's energy pull has ceased.

SHADES OF CRYSTALS

Some crystals come in every shade and type of shading you can imagine: red ones, orange ones, etc. The tones do not yet indicate their recovery or vibrational capacity, and there are no references for shading. There are numerous different kinds of crystals and gemstones out there, and new ones are being made constantly. For shading references for crystals that are more than one tone, you can either mind the significant shading that is observable or join the credits between the various tones.

Red crystals invigorate, initiate, and stimulate your actual body. Some of them offer security and mental fortitude too. The red shading is associated with the root chakra and aids in the use of reasonable skills and actual stamina.

Orange crystals are made by mixing red and yellow, which brings together the vitality of the red tone and the stability of the yellow tone. The orange color of the sacral chakra shows that it works with the energy flow to control creativity, self-expression, personal power, and confidence.

Yellow crystals are excellent for motivation, centering, happiness, and fulfillment issues. This tone is associated with the Solar Plexus Chakra and aids in the ability to separate and differentiate in our physical and spiritual lives, as well as in focusing on issues!

Green crystals are commonly referred to as healing stones, but this is not limited to the color green. This tone is related to the heart chakra and chips away at issues of feelings, connections, flourishing, equilibrium, love, and personal space!

Blue crystals are, for the most part, known for all types of correspondence and are related to the throat chakra. Additionally, they turn out magnificently for cleansing, quieting feelings, and articulation issues.

Purple and violet crystals have a magic sort of value about them. They are related to the Third Eye Chakra and manage getting, instinct, and harmony. In addition to motivation, a creative mind, subliminal effects, and a rebalancing of limits, this tone possesses other notable characteristics.

White and transparent crystals are typically associated with the Crown Chakra. These offer credits for clearness, purging, cleaning, and clairvoyant capacities.

Dark crystals retain the light. They are related to establishing a negative reputation, discretion, and insurance issues. The Omega Chakra is attributed to this tone and its related properties.

Pink crystals have delicate and relieving properties. They are associated with the Heart Chakra as the subsequent tone and energy base. Their properties and ample assistance help manage adoration and goals.

Multi-shaded crystals are fundamental in explicit crystal families. Their color matches depend on how the tones are mixed together and how strong each tone is.

CRYSTAL AND CHAKRA CORRESPONDENCES

Crystal correspondences with the chakras are straightforward and simple to employ. Chakras are recognized as energy centers located throughout our bodies that keep vital energy flowing! In our etheric fields, there are seven main chakras, more than 300 small chakras, and many rose chakras.

Each chakra has a corresponding tone and its own properties. When you add in the properties of the crystals, you can see how crystal healing can put you on a path to healing that seems to come from another world. You don't need to see every crystal and every chakra trait to work with their recovery.

Place the shadow of a suitable crystal or gemstone on or over the chakra region while meditating or participating in a healing session to facilitate chakra recovery and utilization. This will stimulate the chakras, remove any obstructions, and make arrangements possible throughout your energy centers.

Feet Chakras: Minor chakras are located in the arch of each foot. Agate, brown calcite, brown carnelian, and chalcedony quartz are best used for this chakra.

Omega Chakra: Minor Chakra Located beneath your Root Chakra, between your thighs, in your etheric energy fields. Onyx, Obsidian, Hematite, and Black Tourmaline are best used for this chakra.

Root Chakra: Major chakra; located at the base of your spine. Red Jasper, Ruby, Garnet, and Lodestone are best used for this chakra.

Sacral Chakra: Major Chakra. Located just beneath your navel or tummy button. Carnelian, Orange Jasper, Citrine, and Topaz are best used for this chakra.

Hand Chakras: Minor chakras, located in the palms of each hand. You can use any crystal you feel attracted to when working with your hand chakras, as they will hold your crystals. You can generally work with a Clear Quartz for this chakra on the off chance that you are struggling to settle on a choice. Continuously trust your instinct when deciding on your crystal!

Sun-oriented Plexus Chakra: Major Chakra: Located over the navel and underneath your rib cage. Yellow Calcite, Yellow Jasper, Amber, and Tiger's Eye are best used for this chakra.

Spleen Chakra: Minor chakra; located under the left armpit region. Rhodochrosite, Emerald, and Jade are best used for this chakra. This chakra territory can be a possible site for energy spillage.

Heart Chakra: Major Chakra Positioned in the center of your chest. Aventurine, Malachite, and Jade are best used for this chakra.

Higher Heart Chakra: Minor Chakra: Located simply over the heart chakra focus Rose Quartz and Rhodonite are best used for this chakra. A green and pink blend is most appropriate for the heart, and the higher heart chakras are joined to make a passionate base for clearing.

Throat Chakra: is a Major chakra located at the base of the throat. Lapis Lazuli, Sodalite, Turquoise, and Aquamarine are the best stones for this chakra.

Previous existence Chakra: Minor chakra is located simply behind the ear. Blue Fluorite, Amazonite, Amber, and Angelite are best used for this chakra.

Third Eye Chakra: Major Chakra—located between the brows in the center of the forehead. Amethyst, Iolite, Fluorite, and Tanzanite are best used for this chakra.

Soma Chakra: Minor chakra; located simply over the Third Eye Chakra. Amethyst, Charoite, Solid Purple Fluorite, and Purple Quartz (not to be mistaken for Amethyst) are the best stones for this chakra.

Crown Chakra: Major chakra; located simply over the middle and top of the head. Clear Quartz, Herkimer Diamond, and White Amethyst are best used for this chakra.

Higher Crown Chakra: Etheric Chakra, located simply over the Crown Chakra. Stilbite, Sugilite, Pink Topaz, and Zircon are best used for this chakra.

CRYSTAL AND AURA CORRESPONDENCES

Each human, plant, animal, and other living thing possesses a unique quality. Your quality is the electromagnetic field that encompasses your actual body. The atmosphere comprises seven levels, each with its own exciting recurrence. They are interconnected and influence each other through our emotions, feelings, thoughts, actions, wellbeing, and much more. When one of the bodies is out of balance, it makes the other bodies feel awkward.

When we have cynicism issues, stagnant energy, and different issues, they can show up inside our emanation fields before they can affect us inside our actual body. They show up in the auric area as breaks, tears, stagnant energy, and energy engravings. To work with recovering these zones and issues, you need to realize which fitting crystal can work the best for each level to get to the foundation of the issue. Their shading does not relate to the crystals, as it does with chakra healings; they are used for each level, however, because of their recovering properties and qualities.

To use crystals for quality issues, place the crystals in your dominant hand and make enormous clearing movements as far around you as could be expected. Make sure you use the right crystals and crystal stones for the right layer to help fix problems and get rid of old and bad fuel sources.

Atmosphere Alignment: Use Citrine to help adjust your airfields.

Quality Booster: Use Sugilite to give your emanation handle an increase in energy.

Quality Cleanser: Use Lapis Lazuli to give an overall essential purifying.

Air Protection: Use Labradorite to ensure and pad your essential quality requirements.

Air Mood and Opening: Use Rutilated Quartz to improve your temperament and open your atmosphere.

First Auric Level: This is known as your actual emanation body, and it shows your real sensations. Use Lepidolite or Jasper to scrub and mend your first level.

Second Auric Level: This is known as your "etheric quality body" and shows feelings regarding oneself. Use Angelite or Rhyolite to purify and mend your subsequent levels.

Third Auric Level: This is called your level-headed mind, and it tries to help you understand a situation clearly and wisely. Use Aventurine or Bloodstone to cleanse and heal your third level.

Fourth Auric Level: This is known as your astral or passionate body. This level of arrangement fits with our caring cooperation with loved ones. Use Peridot or Rose Quartz to purge and mend your fourth level.

Fifth Auric Level: This is known as your lower atmosphere body. This level works with the divine energy from inside your spirit and on an otherworldly level. Use Carnelian or Staurolite to purge and mend your fifth level.

6th Auric Level: This is known as your higher mental quality body and shows divine love and profound joy. Use Phenacite or Turquoise to scrub and recuperate your sixth level.

Seventh Auric Level: This is known as your mystical and instinctive quality body. This aids in communicating with the heavenly brain and comprehending the more prominent, all-encompassing example of experiencing stillness. Use Celestite or Elestial to scrub and recover your seventh level.

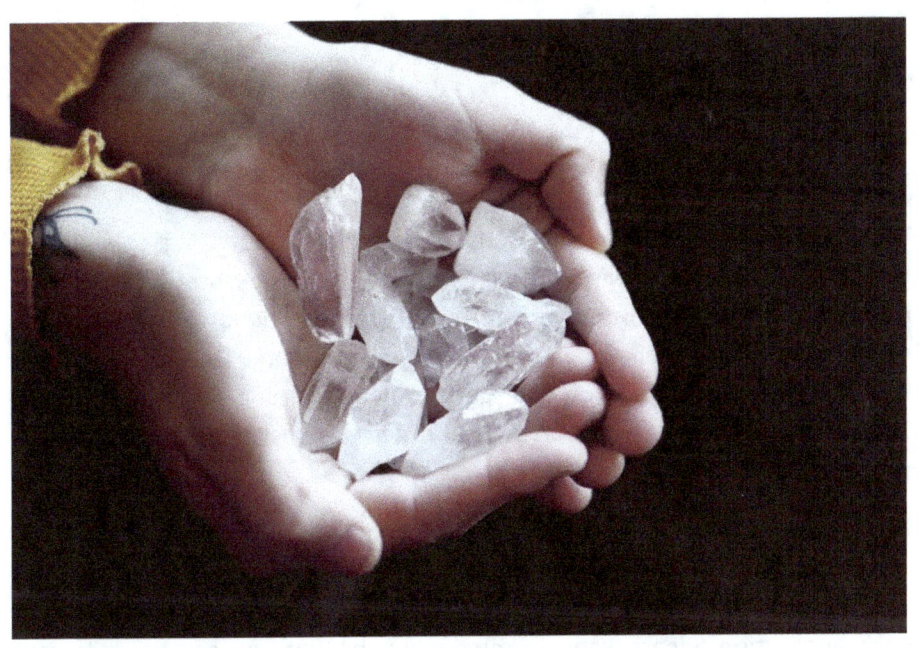

CHAPTER FIVE

HOW TO USE CRYSTALS FOR HEALING.

There are numerous different kinds of approaches to using crystals for recovery. There are likewise various crystals that can be used for different issues and illnesses. I'm not here to reveal that you need to use a specific crystal with a particular goal in mind, or it will not work. That isn't the issue here. I'm here to help you on your path to deep learning and teach you the best ways I've found to use crystals and get the best results for different problems.

As there are numerous ways to use crystals for healing, I have provided an overview of each of the general methods so that you can become proficient with the fundamentals and then apply them to the appropriate crystals for each application. Please keep in mind, though, that you can use different crystals if the ones I've listed don't resonate with your vibrational fields. What makes some of these recovery methods work best is the mix of crystals, the techniques used with them, and how they are used.

WEARING OR CARRYING YOUR CRYSTAL

Putting the crystals in your spiritual fields is probably the easiest way to use them, but is it always the most effective? Some of the time, it is, and once in a while, it isn't. You do have the crystal energy inside your vibrational energy fields. However, on the off chance that you don't put it where you need it the most or leave it there for a sufficiently protracted timeframe, it will just touch the side effects of the affliction and not the source. If you don't keep working with this one crystal until the problem is solved, it can come back, and the cycle starts all over again.

On the other hand, carrying or wearing a crystal can be beneficial if this is something you enjoy doing or wish to do to approach these energies continuously. Simple approaches to doing this are to just carry the crystal in your pocket or handbag, wear the crystal in a pendant package, or use other such adornment plans. This is both trendy and effective!

When working with crystals like this, make sure to eliminate them and scrub them consistently, as they are working with your energetic fields and those you interact with. So make sure to clean and program them regularly, depending on the situation!

CRYSTAL GRIDDING

Crystal gridding is the laying of stones close to the body for healing purposes. This also refers to where crystals are placed in a room or area, such as in meditation circles.

Putting gemstones on someone to help them get better should be possible if the crystal or crystal stone is put close to the right chakra, just as the problem is fixed. You may place the crystal directly on this space or within a few crawls of it. Make sure to use more modest and lighter-weight crystals for this, as they tend to roll and tumble about. If you place the crystal on the correct chakra point and it continues to fall off multiple times, there is a reason! It is, for the most part, because the individual and the crystal are not reverberating inside a similar vibrational match, so pick another proper crystal for this space. This won't occur regularly, yet when it does, it is for an explanation, so watch the healing meeting and how it comes to pass!

The position of crystals inside a room or region is a basic cycle. For the current issue, ensure that the crystals are placed within the space to invest the most energy. For some, it very well might be the parlor, family room, or even the kitchen. The crystal should be set up in the room in such a way that it can reach a full range of fiery vibrations without being stopped. Please do not wrap them in pads and covers, place them in a case, and store them in a trunk in the storage room. They won't have lively access. Setting them toward the sides of the room gives, for the most part, the best access to most of the rooms; however, again, everything depends upon what you are using them for. So if it's not too much trouble, follow the rules per issue to help manage you to the best situation for your room or region.

Reflection circles are consistently fun and a simple strategy for everybody to use. During your reflection meeting, these are basically the circles of your crystals or gemstones that go around your body. You create an image of solidarity with them by placing them all around you. This picture doesn't start or end, so the energy is always moving through each crystal in your energy fields. During your contemplation meeting, this is where the powers are at their most important level. Make sure to scrub and program them consistently.

CRYSTAL ELIXIRS

Crystal elixirs are a water-based base of the crystal's credits, including its healing properties and the programming or purpose behind them to aid in healing. The charged water would then be sprayed on the affected area, used to moisten the area, or poured all over to clean and do other things.

There are numerous approaches to making crystal elixirs. I, for one, have three favorite methods of using them. With so many different routes out there for charging and creating a solution, please try them all and see which ones are most appropriate for you! Kindly use packaged or spring water for making your elixirs, not faucet water, because of its added compounds. Make a point to cover and store your charged crystal remedy water in the cooler, and keep it for as long as seven days.

Direct crystal charging is done when your crystal is submerged in water. Ensure that you have cleaned and customized your appropriate crystal in advance. Empty the water measure into a glass compartment and tenderly spot your crystal in the water. Leave your crystal in the water for the shortest period of time recommended for that particular remedy. Delicately eliminate the crystal and flush, dry, and store this in an uncommon spot.

Aberrant Crystal Charge is done along these lines; however, as opposed to being submerged in the water, you will put your crystal close to your glass water holder. This is a great strategy to use for crystals that can be harmful if ingested.

Crystal Within Charge is a more confusing version of ICC (Indirect Crystal Charge). However, I have discovered it to be more effective when making elixirs. To do this, you will require two glass bowls, one more modest than the other. In your more modest glass bowl, place your scrubbed and customized crystal. Next, place your more modest bowl inside your larger glass bowl. Fill your extra-large glass bowl with bottled or spring water immediately. Your crystal shouldn't touch the water, but it should be surrounded by it, all other things being equal. After your good period has passed, discard your crystal and replace it with a smaller glass bowl, then pour the water from your larger glass bowl into your capacity holder.

ESSENTIAL CRYSTAL HEALING BAGS

When you initially get into crystal recovery, it tends to be confusing, as there are so many crystals and crystal stones out there and just as many reasons and approaches to using them. It is excellent to begin with the basics and trim, so you can start working from that point. This way, you won't become overly overwhelmed by the sheer number of options available to you.

You will need to assemble your own crystal healing units or packs. I think you should get at least two similar crystals for each of the seven chakras that are connected to the seven main principles, as well as any other crystals or gemstones that you feel drawn to on your way to the other side. Some acceptable general recovery stones are explicitly for men, ladies, youngsters, and pets that you can keep close by. This way, when a crisis comes up, you will probably have a portion of the fundamental crystals effectively under your ownership and won't have to stress over rushing to your closest comprehensive store only for a specific crystal or stone. Some real crystals to stock in a crystal recovery pack or unit for anyone are:

Functional Crystal Healing

Red Colored Crystals: Red Jasper or Garnet

Orange Colored Crystals: Carnelian or Topaz

Yellow Colored Crystals: Tiger's eye or Calcite

Green Colored Crystals: Green Aventurine or Emerald

Blue Colored Crystals: Turquoise or Lapis Lazuli

Purple/Violet Colored Crystals: Amethyst or Fluorite

Pink Colored Crystals: Rose Quartz or Rhodonite

White/Clear Colored Crystals: Clear Quartz Crystals or Moonstone

Dark Colored Crystals: Onyx or Black Tourmaline

These are some acceptable staples to have in a crystal healing pack or sack, like gauze and anti-toxin wash in a medical aid unit. Now, you can add crystals of different sizes and shapes to your crystal units or bags, but you always need to have the "essentials" handy!

Some fine crystals and crystal stones turn out better for specific sorts of energy, like male energy, female energy, kids' energy, and creative energy. These are extraordinary items to have on hand, particularly if you intend to consistently work with crystals and their energies.

Some top male energy crystals and crystal stones are: Amethyst, Garnet, Jade, Rose Quartz, Smoky Quartz, Hematite, Malachite, and Lapis Lazuli

Some top female energy crystals and crystal stones are Amber, Amethyst, Jasper, Rose Quartz, Moonstone, Jade, Obsidian, and Sodalite.

Essential Crystal Healing Bags

Some top kids' energy crystals and crystal stones are Amethyst, Apache Tear, Carnelian, Clear Quartz, Rose Quartz, Lapis Lazuli, Tiger's Eye, and Aventurine.

Some top creature energy crystals and gemstones are Amethyst, Rose Quartz, Smoky Quartz, Clear Quartz, Turquoise, Calcite, Carnelian, and Sodalite.

These are great crystals and gemstones to add to your crystal recovery pack or sack, especially if you work with a certain kind of energy. For example, if you want to work with animals, try to stay close to crystals that will help you quickly and effectively balance the energy of your animal friend.

Crystals and Gemstones Alphabetical Index

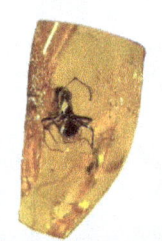 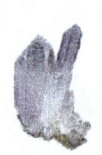 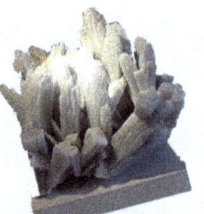

AMBER AMETHYST ANGELITE

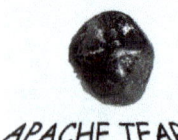 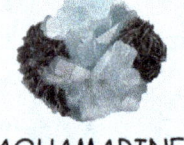

APACHE TEARS AQUAMARINE ARAGONITE

 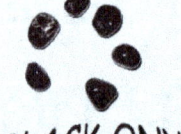 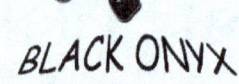

AZURITE BLACK ONYX BLACK TOURMALINE

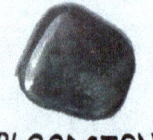 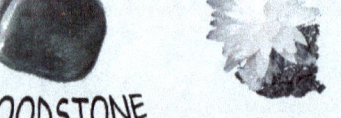 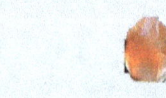

BLOODSTONE CALCITE CRYSTAL CARNELIAN

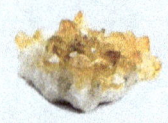 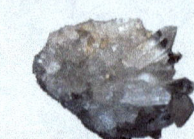 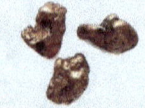

CITRINE CLEAR QUARTZ COPPER STONE

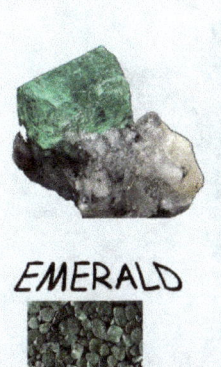 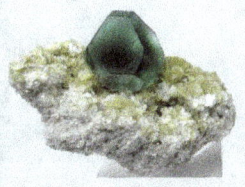 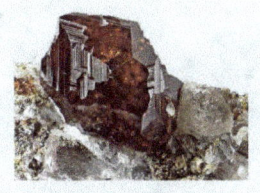

EMERALD FLUORITE GARNET

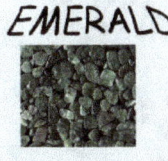 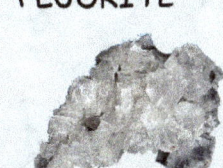 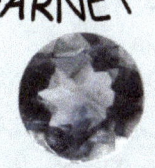

GREEN A. VENTURINE HALITE IOLITE.

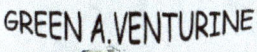 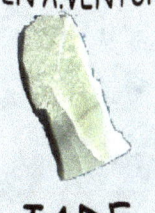 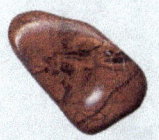 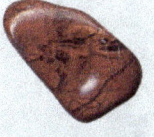 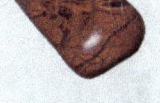 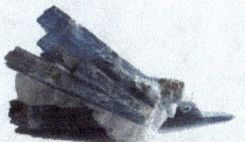

JADE JASPER KYANITE

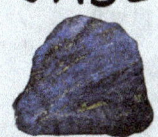 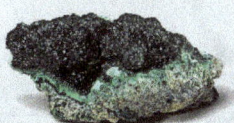 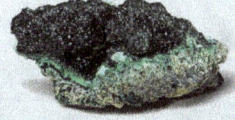 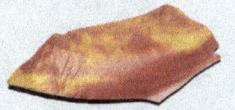

LAPIS LAZULI MALACHITE MOOKAITE

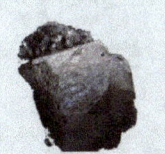 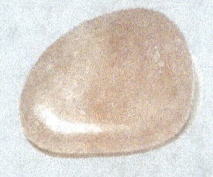 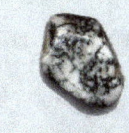

MOONSTONE MORGANITE MOSSAGATE

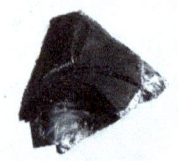 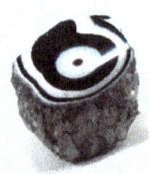 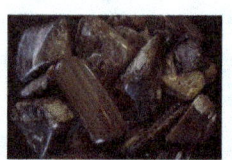

OBSIDIAN   ONYX   PETRIFIED WOOD

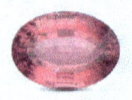 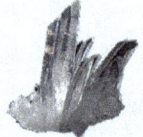 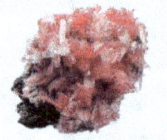

TOURMALINE   QUARTZ   RHODONITE.

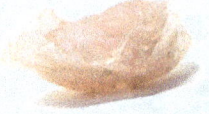 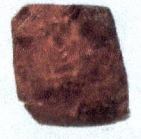 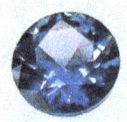

ROSE QUARTZ   RUBY   SAPPHIRE

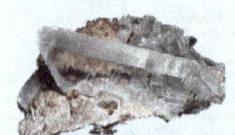 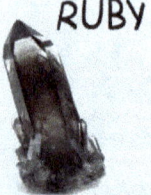 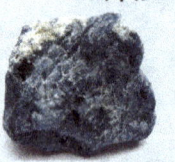

SELENITE   SMOKY QUARTZ   SODALITE

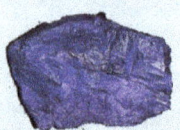 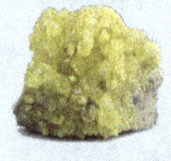 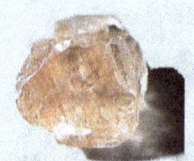

SUGILITE   SULFUR   SUNSTONE

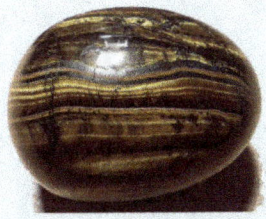

TIGER'S EYE

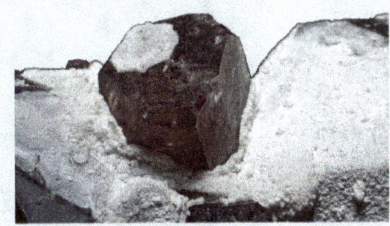

TOPAZ

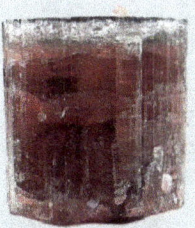

TOURMALINE

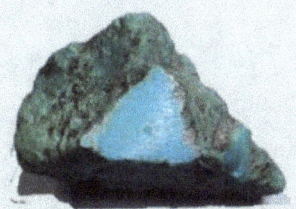

TURQUOISE

CHAPTER SIX

CRYSTAL HEALING TIPS AND TECHNIQUES

Relinquishment:

For five days, wear a rhodonite crystal as close as you can get to your heart chakra to help with deserting.

Mid-region:

Lie down and place two Smoky Quartz crystals, one on each side of your mid-region, and one straight in the middle. Unwind and inhale gradually for 20 minutes, allowing agony and strain to die down.

Scraped spots:

Make a carnelian and black obsidian diamond mixture, charge for 60 minutes, and tenderly pat or fog the territory as regularly as possible on a case-by-case basis.

Plenitude:

Make an Emerald Pearl solution, charge it for 24 hours, and tenderly fog all spaces in your home, office, or wherever you wish to have more bounty in your life.

Misuse Issues:

Sit surrounded by substituted rhodochrosite, emerald, and rose quartz. Record on a piece of paper everything you feel about the present circumstance. Request comprehension and harmony to proceed onward with your life. Cover your paper with Mother Earth. Scrub your crystals altogether a while later.

Acknowledgement:

Putting charoite in the four corners of the room where you spend the most time and energy will bring recognition into your life.

Accomplish Goals:

Place a clear quartz crystal with the sharp end facing straight at yourself when zeroing in and focusing on this objective.

Heartburn:

Make sure to wear a mix of bloodstone and smokey quartz in a pendant for a reduction in manifestations. Each evening, rest with the two stones over your heart chakra for 15 minutes to help recuperate the primary chakra. Purify each evening altogether!

Skin break out:

Make an amethyst pearl solution, charge it for 2 hours, and delicately sprinkle your face with this water two times each day.

Dynamic ENERGY ISSUES:

Carry a red jade inside your quality fields with you for five days to upgrade these issues.

ADHD:

Put a green jade armband on the person's dominant wrist and a black onyx anklet on their lower leg to change the energy in their auras.

Attestations / Mantras:

Hold rhodonite in the middle of your hands when saying your affirmations or mantras; each is an ideal opportunity for seven days to upgrade their capacity.

Forcefulness:

Rub a blue tourmaline quickly to get a positive and negative charge on the ends. Next, put the positive end close to the person or thing that is causing trouble, and the positive harmony energy will spread out to create peace and quiet.

Air Energy:

Carry or wear a blue lace agate to improve air vibrations for seven days.

Air Purifier:

Make a Clear Quartz Crystal Jewel remedy, charge it for 2 hours, and gently fog the air and zones you need to decontaminate.

Plane Ear:

For the torment and pressing factor when flying, try to use a fluorite and black tourmaline blend, turning counterclockwise inside two crawls of the ear until ear agony and the pressing element die down.

Akashic Records:

To get to your Akashic Records more easily, place a crystal network of five Chinese writing stones around you during contemplation. Spot one in front, one behind, and one on each side of your actual body, and hold the final remaining one in your dominant hand during your meeting.

Arrangement:

Lie down and place three citrine crystals around your actual body. Spot one at your feet, one at your mid-region, and one at your crown chakra for 15 minutes.

Sensitivities:

Make a carnelian jewel mixture, charge it for 2 hours, and delicately fog your whole body from your head to your toes up to three times each day.

Enhance CRYSTAL HEALING:

Use phenacite to boost the healing power of other crystals when working with them in recovery meetings. Holding phenacite in your dominant hand and the crystal you're using for that meeting in your other hand will produce the best results.

Butt-centric FISSURES:

Take a relaxing shower in charged shower water of carnelian and golden topaz. Charge the bathwater for 10 minutes prior to your shower. Rehash as frequently as possible on a case-by-case basis.

Scientific Issues:

Carry a purple quartz crystal for five days to see the difference in energy arrangement for this issue.

Heavenly messenger COMMUNICATION:

During contemplation meetings, put Angelite in a full circle around you and watch your relationship improve.

Outrage:

Hold a Blue Lace Agate and take moderate, full breaths. Feel your feet connecting to Mother Earth and all of your anger leaving your body and being turned back into sound energy. It requires around 5 minutes to be quiet and calm once more!

Pets Communication:

Make sure to wear faden quartz when working with creature correspondence to improve the association.

Pets Injury:

Take a rose quartz and spot this inside a couple of creeps of the creature's physical issue. Turn the crystal clockwise to help this draw move the stuck and negative energy from the injury out of the body. Keep an eye out for negative reactions from the creature. They can't use crystal energy as quickly as people can, so it would be best to tone it down.

Pets Protection:

Place angelite on your pet's case or their collar for additional insurance for their energy fields.

Tension:

Hold the peridot in your dominant hand and rub it delicately with your thumb. You can likewise put this over your heart chakra and inhale gradually and profoundly. Your tension level will drop within a couple of moments.

Appreciation:

Use this on yourself by conveying or wearing Howlite inside your energy fields for at least three days to see the energy shifts change significantly. To chip away at appreciation issues with others, place two in the inverse corners of the room where they invest the most energy for at least 14 days and see the adjustment of conduct.

Contention:

During a contention, get your hematite and tenderly hold it in the middle of your hands. Gradually breathe out the entirety of your breath, delicately blowing over the hematite. Put your hands down and take the hematite in the hand you use most. Take a few moments to relax to calm the raised issues.

Pomposity Issues:

Carry or wear an Emerald for seven days to manage self-image and self-importance issues.

Joint inflammation:

Make a carnelian-jewel mixture, charge it for three hours, and wash your hands in this water to ease the agony. You can likewise apply the water directly to the affected region.

Climb:

Hold a little White Spirit Quartz, one in each hand, during your contemplation meetings to build up your rising capacities.

Decisive:

Carry an Amazonite with you when you should be more confident, for example, when you are busy working, to raise your vibration level.

ASTHMA:

For individuals who suffer from asthma, wear a Tiger's Eye pendant low enough on a chain to be as near your lungs as could be expected. The energy vibration will help quiet the problems you're facing and cut down on the attacks.

ASTRAL ENERGY CORD REMOVAL:

Use Variscite when working with astral energy line expulsion meetings. Make sure to hold this in your predominant hand when chipping away at pulling the energy strings, and use this vibrational-level energy to help them seal shut.

ASTRAL PROJECTION:

Place hematite in a circle around you before you start your meeting, or hold one in your dominant hand when your meeting starts!

ASTRAL TRAVEL:

Geodes are magnificent for working with astral travel and come in different structures like quartz, amethyst, citrine, and calcite. When you're having a meeting about astral travel, you should make sure to surround yourself with as many geodes as could be expected under the circumstances. Ensure they are overall similar in color. Clear quartz and amethyst are magnificent stones to use for this reason.

ATHLETE'S FOOT:

Soak your feet in charged water of Emerald and Smoky Quartz. Make sure to purge the crystals after every meeting.

Air Alignment:

During an air meeting, combine citrine into the healing to help balance the energies and adjust them to the actual body.

Atmosphere Booster:

Wear Sugilite to ingest negative energy from inside your airways. Make sure to purge each last day of wearing once more!

Emanation Cleaner:

Use a lapis lazuli during your purifying meeting and circumvent the customer's quality fields, sending energy to heal any tears, openings, stagnant, or negative energy. Make sure to purge the crystal after the meeting.

Emanation Opening:

Use a rutilated quartz during a quality meeting to create a more open and open atmosphere.

Mental imbalance:

Make sure to put Charoite around the spaces where the medically introverted individual invests the most energy to help quiet down the issues they are managing inside.

AUTOMOBILE TRAVEL:

Make sure to put a moonstone in your vehicle's trunk and one in the glove box when traveling. If you are traveling by bike or car, make a point to put one in the vehicle's compartment.

Mindfulness:

Carry or wear a pendant of celestite, have this in a typical space in your home or office, and even use this in reflection meetings to open up your mindfulness.

Back Problems:

For a short beginning eruption of distress, it rests on your stomach and has somebody place three bits of petrified wood on your back, similarly far off from the scruff of your neck to your tailbone. Rest for 15 minutes, and your back agony will be soothed. For consistent issues, wear an opposite pendant, so the petrified wood is laying on your back, not your chest, for six hours per day for five days in a row. The issues will be diminished in seriousness.

Terrible Breath:

Make a carnelian and onyx diamond mixture, charge for 15 minutes, and flush orally as frequently as needed on a case-by-case basis.

Adjusting the Physical and Spiritual Worlds:

Carry Moldavite around with you on these occasions to reestablish the harmony between the physical and otherworldly universes.

Balancer:

Onyx is an overall body balancer. Spot this in a pendant around your neck to reestablish harmony throughout your whole body.

Bed Sores:

Make a turquoise and black tourmaline jewel solution, charge it for 20 minutes, and douse a cotton ball in the remedy. Depending on the situation, you can pat the sores with the charged water on the cotton ball that has been wet.

Bedwetting Issues:

Place a golden topaz in two inverse corners of the bed edge and a carnelian in the other two inverse corners of the bed edge to help settle bed-wetting issues.

Conduct Issues:

For the best behavior, have the person wear a tiger's eye on their dominant hand and the lower leg on the other side.

Bipolar Disorder:

To help counteract erratic bipolar turmoil issues, make sure you wear a combination of turquoise, rose quartz, and onyx. Onyx is best worn around your lower legs for a winning combination, while turquoise and rose quartz are best worn around your wrists or hands.

Bladder Trouble:

Lie down and place two amber pieces, one on each side of your hips. Allow the energy to flow and rest for 20 minutes.

Bulging When swelling:

happens, it rests on three golden topazes and spots every one of them over your stomach/midsection territory in a triangle shape. Ensure you make them point close to your crown chakra and the other two under this main one, framing a triangle shape. Rest and unwind for 15 minutes. Rehashing depends on the situation, and scrub the stones thoroughly when the meeting is finished.

Obstructed ROOT CHAKRA:

Hold the lodestone within four crawls of the root chakra and move it around in a clockwise direction to clear any blockages. Make sure to scrub entirely after that.

Impeded SACRAL CHAKRA:

Place carnelian on each side of the sacral chakra, and hold citrine inside four crawls of the chakra and go clockwise to eliminate any blockages. Make sure to purge altogether subsequently.

Obstructions to the solar plexus chakra:

Place Yellow Jasper on each side of the sun-oriented plexus chakra and hold Clear Quartz inside four crawls of the chakra, and go clockwise to eliminate any blockages. Make sure to scrub altogether a while later.

Impeded Heart Chakra:

Place a rose quartz on each side of the heart chakra, hold moldavite inside the four corners of the chakra, and go clockwise to eliminate any blockages. Make sure to purify altogether after that

Third Eye Chakra:

Place fluorite on each side of the third eye chakra, hold prehnite inside the four corners of the chakra, and go clockwise to eliminate any blockages. Make sure to purify altogether subsequently.

Hinged Crown Chakra:

Hold danburite in the four corners of the crown chakra and move it around in a clockwise motion to clear out any blockages. Make sure to purge for a short time and completely later.

Hindered Feet Chakra:

Hold hematite inside four of the foot chakras and go clockwise to eliminate any blockages. Make sure to purge altogether a short time later.

Obstrufluorite Chakras:

Place an amethyst on each side of the hand chakra and hold a clear quartz inside four crawls of the hand chakra, then run your energy, pulling from a universal source to eliminate any blockages. Make sure to purge completely subsequently.

Poor Blood Circulation:

Wear a citrine pendant, just as wristbands and anklets do, to assist with the association and stream!

Circulatory strain Wear or convey a mix of black and green tourmaline around with you to reliably offset these issues.

Red Eyes:

Make a mixture of clear quartz crystal and emerald, charge it for 60 minutes, and spot a couple of drops of the charged water in each eye. Rehash as required.

Vent:

Hold one red jade in each hand, focus on the issues that are bubbling up inside, and take three profound, sluggish relaxations. Ensure you scrub them thoroughly after each use.

Self-perception Issues:

If you have problems with how you see yourself, wear a smokey quartz necklace and anklet at the same time to turn these problems around and see yourself in a good and holy light.

Holding Issues:

Place jade and rose quartz in the inverse corners of the room, where the individual invests the most energy. These energies will help them bond faster.

BONES:

Make a mixture of fluorite pearls, let it sit for 24 hours, and then lightly fog it on the bone area you want to strengthen. You can also take a shower and let the water charge for 10 minutes before you get in. This will help raise your vibrational level and strengthen your bones.

BONE LOSS:

Wear rhodonite 24 hours per day for six days straight. At that point, scrub for one day. Rehashing depends on the situation.

Limit Issues:

Make sure you program and convey Barite with you to places where you encounter limit issues, for example, work or a relative's home. Convey this as regularly as is conceivable when at the areas, and purify after every meeting.

Internal Issues:

Use yellow jasper in a recovering meeting to assist in quieting issues with the inside inconvenience. Use three of them during the session: one on each side of the customer and one over their lower midsection.

Brainwaves:

When you meditate, rest, or sleep with a Herkimer Diamond near your head, your brainwave frequency and subliminal perceptions will be more in sync.

Breaking ties:

Use Onyx to acclimate to issues involving breaking ties. Wear one around your lower leg and one around your dominant wrist for seven days. Make sure to scrub them after that!

Broken Heart:

Use green aventurine and rose quartz together to patch a messed-up heart. Rest for 15 minutes and spot the two stones over your heart chakra. When you get up, envelop them with a piece of paper and cover them in your lawn for five days. Make sure to uncover them after the five days and tenderly purge them.

Wounds:

Make a solution of petrified wood and hematite pearls, let it charge for two hours, and then fog or pat the injured area, depending on what you need to do.

BUNIONS:

Wear an anklet made of carnelian and smokey quartz to get rid of the energy blockage in that area, which is the main cause of your bunions.

Weights:

Carry Amber around with you in your pocket or tote to help facilitate the issues with loads. For a more grounded association, have this with you 24 hours per day for three days to reduce the weight.

Consumes:

Make a chrysoprase solution, charge the water for 60 minutes, and tenderly pat the region required with this charged water. You can likewise add drops of this to some other cure, cream, or salve you do use for different recovering purposes.

BUSINESS/CAREER:

Take malachite in the middle of your hands and focus on your business achievements and what you need to have changed or occur. Spot the malachite in your tote or close to your wallet for five days after this, and watch your business dreams show!

Quieting the Body:

Lie down and encircle yourself with blue topaz and agate for 15 minutes to feel your actual body quiet down!

Quieting the Mind:

Lie down and place agate and amethyst over your third eye chakra, and take them in profoundly. Take 10 minutes, and your brain will be quiet, loose, and revived!

Disease:

Use selenite in a recovering crystal meeting for issues with malignant growth. Do a total healing session from head to toe using selenite. Make sure to scrub the stone completely subsequently.

Carpel Tube:

Make a blue-lace agate pearl mixture, charge it for three hours, and wash your hands in this water to facilitate the torment. You can likewise straightforwardly apply the water to the affected territory.

Cell Healing Program:

Use an elestial quartz during a phone recovery meeting to intensify its effectiveness.

Cell Memory:

Use a citrine herkimer to upgrade your cell's memory. No matter what the meeting is about, make sure you have this with you, either all around you or in the hand you use most.

Cell Renewal:

Take six mochi balls and rest on your back. Have two put at your feet, one on each side of you, one at your crown chakra, and one on your mid-region. Inhale deeply and slowly, and take in all the energy you'll need for 20 minutes at once. Rehash until desired outcomes appear.

Cellulite:

Make a diamond remedy of hematite and golden topaz, charge it for 60 minutes, and delicately fog all regions where cellulite appears. Rehash it multiple times every day.

Focusing:

For focusing practice, hold a yellow topaz close to your sun-powered plexus chakra and place a black phantom quartz at your feet. Take it in gradually and profoundly for 10 minutes.

CHAKRAS BALANCED:

To adjust your chakras, take seven crystals (one for each chakra's color correspondence) and lie on your back. Spot the corresponding crystals in alignment with your chakras for 20 minutes. Make sure to purge them all exclusively after the meeting. To intensify the engagement, encircle yourself with four clear quartz crystals. One at your feet, one on each side of your body, and one at your crown chakra. Ensure the transparent quartz crystals are, for the most part, pointing inward!

CHAKRA ENERGY FLOW:

Place an elestial crystal at your crown chakra in the wake of finishing a chakra adjustment meeting. Rest and unwind, appreciating the new, more grounded energy stream, for 15 minutes!

CHAKRAS OPENED:

Opening a shut chakra should be possible with fluorite placed on top of the chakra while resting. Turn the fluorite clockwise multiple times. If the chakra is as yet shut, do another meeting until it is open and streaming normally.

Change:

Use purple rainbow fluorite to help you get through changes and get out of the trenches as much as possible. During this timeframe, scrub this day by day.

Change your perspective:

Hold one clear calcite crystal in your dominant hand and spotlight the theme for 10 minutes. Heft this around with you for the following few days and witness the progress from your own perspective.

Diverting Ability:

Surround yourself with Sugilite before your meeting starts, or grasp them before beginning a directing meeting. Others have even laid down with them under their cushions to build their associations!

Bedlam:

Hold your Tanzanite close to your solar plexus chakra and take deep breaths when things are going wrong.

Liveliness:

Place a Watermelon Tourmaline in the space where you invest the most energy and watch your disposition improve!

Chicken Pox:

Make a chicken pox remedy with black tourmaline, carnelian, and golden topaz to help with the itching and tingling. Charge for 1 hour and delicately fog from head to toe as regularly as necessary, depending on the situation.

Labor:

Use a moonstone to help soothe youngster birthing issues by wearing it as a pendant or having this near you during the birthing cycle. It will quiet you and your child during this new experience!

CHILLS:

Make an aragonite diamond solution and charge it for three minutes. Eliminate the crystals and warm the water. Spot a perfect towel in the charged water and ring out an abundance. Wrap this ludicrous head or neck.

Ongoing Fatigue:

Make sure you wear a Green Phantom Quartz to help battle the issues of managing constant weakness. Make sure to purify this once every other day.

CLAIR AUDIENCE:

Use Snowflake Obsidian by keeping them as near your actual ears as you can. They are not to help your actual ears but rather your inward hearing feeling. You can likewise put them under your cushion when you rest, get studs made of them, or attach them to headsets. The prospects are interminable!

Perceptiveness:

For dealing with creating special insight, use Hawk's Eye in contemplation and directing meetings. You can make a circle of them around yourself, hold one in your dominant hand, or wear one as a pendant to improve your visionary skills and reach your full potential.

Lucidity:

Using Rainforest Jasper does something amazing for this office! Tell your Rainforest Jasper your issues you are befuddled about and need lucidity on. At that point, haul this around with you during seasons of disarray, and inside the space of a few days, normally hours, the disarray is gone and clarity is reestablished.

Scrub CARPET TOXINS:

Make sure you place malachite on each side of the space to purify and cover poisons. Purify the malachite after seven days.

Purging Organs:

Lie down and place five yellow jasper stones around your body. One at your crown chakra, one on each side of your body, one at your feet, and one over your mid-region. Unwind and inhale profoundly for 15 minutes.

Clearing:

Sit down in a chair, and have somebody take a Topaz crystal and gradually work over your emanation layers and energy fields with this crystal. Whenever this is done, make sure to purify the topaz!

Ungainliness:

Using copper is an effective method to assist with awkwardness. You can discover that copper armbands and anklets work the best. But adding a clear quartz pendant to a copper chain necklace also makes for a great combination.

COLIC:

For colic issues, hold a Rhodonite inside 2 crawls of the infant's waist and turn clockwise multiple times like clockwork to settle their energy fields and colicky behavior.

Mouth blisters:

Make a carnelian and turquoise diamond solution, charge it for 60 minutes, and douse a cotton ball in the mixture. Tenderly spot the blister with the doused cotton ball. Use a new, clean cotton ball for every application.

Basic Cold:

For the regular cold, use a yellow topaz to alleviate the symptoms. Charge the bathwater for 10 minutes with this stone and wash up. You can also rest with this stone around your head and another one over your third eye chakra to feel even better.

Solace:

Hold and concentrate with gold calcite while requiring extra soothing energies. This stone will pull your old energy out of you and send it to the universe while giving you new energy to help you rethink things.

Correspondence:

If you wear an aquamarine as a pendant as close as you can to your throat chakra, it will help you get back into balance when it comes to communication.

Correspondence with Plants/Animals:

Find the plant or creature you wish to speak with and hold a fairy stone in your dominant hand. Pose the inquiries you need to think about and sit tight for the appropriate responses. Recall answers can come as sentiments, messages, words, considerations, pictures, and signs, so stay open to the prospects.

Empathy:

Make an Ajoite mixture, charge it for 2 hours, and fog the regions that are deficient with regard to sympathy, regardless of whether it be your home or office, and watch the progressions show up!

Fixation:

Carry or wear a blue topaz on your body to expand your focus levels. On the off chance that you are concentrating in a particular room of your home, make a blue topaz solution, charge for 1 hour, and fog the territory.

Blackout:

When confronted with issues and side effects of a blackout, try to put hematite directly on top of your crown chakra, one in each hand, and one at each foot chakra. Have somebody hold a clear quartz inside two crawls of the third eye chakra and turn it clockwise like clockwork until side effects die down.

Surety:

Carry or wear eudialyte for an increase in additional surety. Program this before wearing to hold the vibrational level.

Struggle:

Place citrine spirit quartz in regions that are feeling a vibrational clash. For the best results, position yourself in the space's inverse corners.

Disarray:

Hold peridot in front of your heart chakra and concentrate on the issues that are bothering you at the time for answers to appear. Rehash in brief timeframe outlines, each lasting only 5 minutes.

Clog:

Lie down and place Aventurine over your lungs, and inhale gradually for 10 minutes. Scrub the stone and rehash it regularly, depending on the situation.

Association (Past and Future):

When working in meetings, make a point to use a blue apatite in your dominant hand or side and a purple apatite in your contrary side to work with past and future associations.

Clogging:

Lie down and place three ajuits around your actual body. Spot one on each side of your lower mid-region and one over the middle. Unwind for 15 minutes for the energy to begin streaming.

Happiness:

Carry or wear Halite for dealing with issues of satisfaction. Make sure to purify the following seven days.

COORDINATION:

Use fluorite to offset excursion coordination issues by carrying it in your pocket. Do this for at least 5 days straight and watch your coordination improve.

CORNS:

Soak your feet in a black onyx jewel remedy that covers the entire foot. In any case, 6 stones for each foot, arranged in a circle around your foot, while dowsing for 15 minutes at a time.

Hacking:

Lie down and place two sodalite crystals, one on each side of your neck territory; place a yellow jasper over your chest region; and spot one clear quartz crystal over your throat chakra. Unwind and gradually relax. You can likewise make a jewel mixture with these crystals, charge it for 60 minutes, and place three drops under your tongue when you begin hacking.

Boldness:

Make an aquamarine and carnelian mixture, charge it for 6 hours, and fog the zones you are most habitually in for this to be the most effective!

Issues:

Lie down and place two hematite, one on each side of the space, and one clear quartz over the space. Unwind and relax. Make sure to purify after every meeting.

Inventiveness:

Surround yourself with amethyst whenever and wherever possible. The more you have, the more vibrational energies for inventiveness will flow. You can think with this, place them all through your home or office, and even fog the territories you are working in with a charged amethyst fog.

Emergency:

Carry or wear a rose quartz pendant during emergency times. You can likewise accuse your bathwater of containing rose quartz and wash up to resolve these issues.

CROHN'S DISEASE:

Rest and place two Clear Quartz on each side of your lower midsection, pointing upwards, and one Smoky Quartz over your navel to alleviate side effects. Unwind for 15 minutes, three times a day, for the manifestations to die down.

Getting Over:

When confronted with a death, try to surround the area with Chiastolite, also known as the Cross Stone, as much as possible to help the spirits get over. You can likewise use this if you have a lost earthbound soul that necessitates help getting over to a meeting to free them from their earthbound ties.

Crying:

Lie down and place a rose quartz over your heart chakra and a smokey quartz on each side of your body. Unwind, cry, and deliver the entirety of the repressed energy. Purify the crystals after every meeting.

Dandruff:

Make a snowflake obsidian and green jade jewel mixture and charge for 60 minutes. After you've washed and rinsed your hair, gently fog this charged water all over your scalp and let it air dry for the best results.

Refusal:

Carry or wear Elestial Quartz for issues requiring disavowal for seven days.

Trustworthy:

Carry a black onyx in each pocket to boost fiery vibrations for stability. If issues are with places or others, make a remedy, charge for 2 hours, and delicately fog all regions that are concerning them.

Despondency:

Use a smoky quartz for gloomy issues by hefting it around in your pocket or wearing it as a pendant.

DERMATITIS:

Make a golden topaz and lapis lazuli diamond mixture, charge it for 60 minutes, and delicately fog all regions that are affected. Rehash on a case-by-case basis.

Depression:

Combine a Green Phantom Quartz and a Rose Quartz to work on issues of despair. Charge and program them before use, and purge them each day.

Commitment:

If you want to focus on how to manage your commitment, put yourself in the middle of a jewel-shaped matrix of garnet and wrap it around you for three minutes every day. Do this for seven days straight, generally at a similar time every day.

Diaper Rash:

Make a mixture of turquoise and clear quartz diamonds, charge it for an hour, and add a few drops of this charged water to the cream or balm you put on the baby's bottom to help them get better much faster!

Looseness of the bowels:

Carry a clear quartz crystal close to your waist, for example, in a pocket or on a belt, to assist quietness and straightforwardness with its recovering vibration!

Trouble SWALLOWING:

Lie down and place a lapis lazuli on each side of your throat chakra, a clear quartz on your throat chakra, and fluorite on your third eye chakra. Rest and unwind for 15 minutes. Scrub your crystals completely and make a diamond remedy of them; charge for 60 minutes; and spot a couple of drops under your tongue a couple of times each day.

Assimilation:

Place Jasper in your pocket for seven days, from morning until evening, and watch how the issues with processing disappear.

Bearing in Life:

Carry White Jade with you, regardless of how much can be reasonably expected during this time! Make a pearl mixture, charge it for three minutes, and gently fog the zones you frequent!

Coordinating Energy:

Place the topaz crystal on top of the situation with the help of an intermediary, such as a letter or a photograph of the individual. On the off chance that this has to do with work issues, place them around your office or on top of your documents. Do this for at least 5 days, and make sure to scrub the crystal subsequently!

Handicaps:

Place amethyst and carnelian around the individual or home that the individual invests the most energy in. This will help to calm the situation and alleviate the stress caused by the inability. Make sure to scrub them once per week!

Disengaged with the Higher Self:

Surround yourself in a circle with clear selenite while reflecting, and your association will be upgraded!

Distance Healing:

During your recovery, combine cobaltite and clear quartz to improve your removed healing meetings.

Dazedness:

Wear a pendant with a clear quartz point during your bleary-eyed spells to help refocus the energies.

DNA Activation:

Use a leopardskin jasper during a DNA enactment meeting to upgrade its effectiveness. Encircle yourself with them or hold one in your dominant hand during the meeting.

Unsureness:

Carry Staurolite in your pocket or wear it as a pendant for full effect on these occasions. After using, make sure to purify!

Dominant Energy:

Keep one Apache Tear in each pocket to acquire more dominant energies while avoiding being exploited to center your energy and become more dominant.

Draw out negative energy.

When you hold Jet in your stronger hand during times of conflict, the energy will flow outward. Make a point of focusing on specific issues and cleaning up after your meeting!

DREAM STIMULATION:

Place citrine under your pad before sleeping if you need more dreams in the evening. Your psyche will showcase your life through your fantasy state!

DREAM RECALL:

If you are now having dreams but need assistance in reviewing them, place a Herkimer Diamond under your pillow before heading to sleep. This will invigorate your memory for review in the first part of the day!

DRY EYES:

Lie down and place an aquamarine over each eye and a clear quartz crystal over your third eye chakra, facing upward for 10 minutes. Rehash on a case-by-case basis.

DRY MOUTH:

Make a Lapis Lazuli and Turquoise Jewel remedy, charge it for three minutes, and then rinse your mouth with the charged water as often as you need to, depending on the situation.

Dyslexia:

To help with dyslexia, have the individual convey or wear Scapolite as much as possible for the best results.

Ear infection;

Lie down on your back, and spot one piece of amber on each side of your head, close to your ears. Unwind and rest for 20 minutes to facilitate the agony.

Earth Energy:

Take Brown Jade with you and stroll outside, shoeless if conceivable, and get back in contact with Mother Earth. Additionally, wear this crystal around your lower leg for more earth energy fascination.

Dermatitis:

Make an Ocean Jasper Pearl remedy, let it sit for an hour, and then fog or pat the areas that need it. On a case-by-case basis, rehash as often as possible.

Effectiveness Faced with efficiency issues:

Carry or wear Limonite in whatever quantity is reasonable for a seven-day period.

ELECTROMAGNETIC ISSUES:

Take two Boji stones, one in each hand, and balance them around the chakras of your palms for 15 minutes to help with electromagnetic problems. Make sure to purify a short time later.

Obstructed Feelings:

Use green tourmaline and rose quartz together to completely deliver your obstructed feelings. Rest and spot these stones over your heart chakra for 15 minutes at a time. Rehash every day until they are totally liberated. Depending on the blockage, this could take anywhere from 1 to 14 days.

Feelings That Need to Be Calmed:

Wear or convey moonstone when your feelings improve. This will help you calm down quickly. Make sure to scrub a short time later.

Sympathy:

When required, rest and spot pink beryl over your heart chakra, then center around the current issue. Unwind and inhale profoundly. Make sure to remain on track during this time.

EMPHYSEMA:

Make a chrysotile diamond remedy, let it sit for two hours, and fog your home, office, and car at regular intervals for 10 days to improve the air quality. Rest for 15 minutes and place a chrysotile over your chest territory and two clear quartz, one on each side of the body pointing upwards, for the actual body. Depending on the situation, repeat as often as possible.

Perseverance:

If you have trouble staying strong, carry sodalite and bloodstone together in your pocket or wear them as a necklace. The blend makes for an additional increase in perseverance when you need it!

Fiery TIES:

If you want to get closer to someone, especially in a romantic way, carry or wear garnet for three days and then put it on the other person's third eye chakra. This will help you connect with them on a deeper level.

Jolt of energy:

Hold two clear quartz crystals, one in each hand, while sitting on a seat with your feet level on the ground. Ensure the sharp edges are pointed toward your body. Inhale gradually and profoundly for 10 minutes for a fast jolt of energy.

ENERGY BALANCE:

When adjusting energies, use two Larimar stones, one in each hand, and sit serenely in a seat. Unwind and ingest the vibrational energies through your hand chakras for 10 minutes.

ENERGY FLOW:

Place albite throughout each chakra in turn, beginning with your crown chakra and working your way down to your first chakra. At that point, do the inverse and work from your root chakra up to your crown chakra. Allow the albite to rest on each chakra for three minutes to allow the energy stream to expand.

ENERGY GRID CLEANSING:

To make an energy matrix purge work better, put ammonite around you or hold it in your dominant hand.

ENERGY IMPRINT REMOVAL:

If you want to get the best results from an energy engraving and expulsion meeting, you should surround yourself with Shaman Phantom Quartz. When playing out an energy engraving and expulsion meeting, make a point to use a Shaman Phantom Quartz in your dominant hand.

ENERGY VAMPIRE:

Make sure you wear amber as a pendant and around your lower leg for the best insurance against energy vampires.

Eagerness:

When you wear or give Fire Agate, your energy level will change and your excitement will go through the roof.

Substance RELEASE WORK:

To commemorate an element releasement meeting, form a circle with charcoal around the customer. Bring the customer's professional and an intermediary if the meeting is held remotely!

Correspondence:

Make a Morganite solution, let it sit for 60 minutes, and then lightly fog all the rooms in your home or office. This will help settle equity issues. Rehash the double-seven days.

Balance:

Lay down and put kyanite on your crown chakra for 15 minutes if you're having trouble getting along with others.

Depletion:

When feeling depleted, put on a Cooper neckband, wristband, or anklet. This additional jolt of energy will pull you out of this vibrational state. Connect a clear crystal to one of them to improve it significantly!

Articulation:

Wear turquoise on a short pendant, as near your throat chakra as could be expected, and notice how your sentiments, feelings, and articulations fire up!

Outer NEGATIVITY:

Wear or carry sodalite inside your energy fields to help keep bad things from happening and to heal them if they do. This can even be done by PCs to reduce EMF harm.

EYES (GENERAL ISSUES):

For eye issues, ensure you have three amethyst crystals and one turquoise stone available. Rest and spot your turquoise at your third eye chakra. The three amethysts ought to be situated, one at your crown chakra and one on each side of your head, in accordance with your eyes. Ensure the amethysts are pointing toward your head. Rest and unwind for 20 minutes.

EYES (CORNEA SCRATCH):

When the eye is closed, place celectite over it and rest for 10 minutes. Place the crystal in two of the eye's corners and turn it clockwise at least a few times to relieve pain and irritation and speed up the healing process.

Swooning:

If you have a lot of blackout spells, wear fluorite as a pendant and turquoise as an arm band as much as you can. This will help your blackout spells be more serious and happen more often.

Pixie REALM ENERGIES:

Use a fairy quartz in your nursery or on your patio to connect with pixie energies more strongly. You can also prepare a diamond mixture, charge it for 60 minutes, and delicately fog the areas outside and inside where you want to have a more profound relationship with these energies.

Decency:

Make a mixture of clear quartz, rose quartz, and tree agate pearls, charge it for 60 minutes, and tenderly fog the individual or territories that are in need of reasonable energy.

Carry or wear an Emerald and Clear Quartz combination to remind you to pull together and stay in the light of acceptance and confidence!

Carry or wear Charoite during these trying times to see how the dismissal problem resolves itself and you can be more open to acting naturally!

FAMILY ISSUES:

Carry or wear a Rainforest Jasper to assist in managing family issues. You can also make a pearl solution, let it sit for an hour, and fog the areas around your house where your family spends the most time.

Dream (CREATE):

Keep Ulexite in your pocket to live a more dream-filled life and communicate your imagination.

Dream (REDUCE): Make sure to wear black obsidian around your throat chakra to lessen dream issues and idealism.

Weariness:

Wear an onyx anklet and a clear quartz crystal pendant to change the vibration.

Dread:

Wear agate on a longer pendant chain near your heart chakra for maximum benefit in dealing with dread issues!

Feet:

For sore or hurting feet, place them in a tub with warm water, ocean salt, 4 black tourmalines, and 1 hematite. Spot the hematite close to the highest point of your toes, two black tourmalines, one on each side of the foot, and the other two black tourmalines back by your impact points. Splash your feet for 15 minutes. Make sure to scrub them after each use.

FEMALE ENERGETIC BALANCE:

Make a pink tourmaline pearl remedy, charge for 2 hours, and fog your whole home or office with this softly, particularly in the corners!

Richness ISSUES:

Carnelian is ideal for problems involving ripeness, fruitlessness, weakness, or periods. Men or women, bring this with you for at least seven days in a row to allow the vibrational healing energy to work to its fullest. On the off chance that issues are with origin and ripeness, make a point to have the carnelian in the four corners of the room to help balance out the energy there too.

FEVER:

To help bring down a fever, make an Agate diamond solution, charge it for 20 minutes, and gently fog the person's crown chakra, hands chakras, and feet chakras at regular intervals. For a more grounded effect, have the individual rest and place hematite at their crown, hands, and feet chakras!

FIBROMYALGIA;

Carry or wear a Tanzine Aura Quartz to help deal with fibromyalgia problems. You can also make a jewel solution, charge it for 2 hours, and use this charged water to gently rub on sore muscles and joints or put it in moisturizers for these problems.

Monetary ISSUES:

The blend of pyrite and green tourmaline functions admirably for making and finding wellsprings of wealth, so you stay open to all that comes in. Make sure to convey or wear them together. You can also keep them in your bag or near your wallet or checkbook for added energy!

Fire Energy:

To have a more grounded association with fire energies, make a point to carry a Fire Agate in your pocket!

Fart:

Flatulence can be a humiliating issue for anyone, so if it becomes more common in your life, keep a Smoky Quartz in your pocket to help you through the times when it occurs. Rest and place two Smoky Quartz, one on each side of your lower mid-region, for day-to-day repair work. Next, place a golden topaz over your navel and two hematites at your foot chakras. Rest and unwind for brief stretches day by day for the best outcomes.

Blossom Energy:

To connect with bloom energies, wrap a fairy cross around your lower leg!

Influenza:

Use a rainforest jasper to aid in the detection of this season's virus. Wear it as a pendant around your neck as much as possible during these occasions.

Liquid Retention:

Place a rainbow moonstone around the spaces that are holding liquids. If this is a damaged area, try to encompass it as much as possible while also placing another on top of the space. Unwind and permit the vibrational energies to labor for 15 minutes all at once.

FLYING ISSUES/STRESS:

Wear a hematite pendant to relieve anxiety and dissatisfaction while also assisting you in making the most of your flight travel.

FOOD CLEANSING:

To get rid of poisons, hold a clear quartz-ended crystal in your dominant hand and slowly turn it clockwise over each piece of food before you eat it. Scrub after each use.

Carelessness/MEMORY:

Carry a mix of Emerald and Howlite around with you, or spot them in your home or office together for the most grounded effect. Make an effort to keep this as close to you as possible, as it will aid in memory restoration.

Absolution:

You can use Sugilite by holding it in your dominant hand and focusing on how to solve a problem. Request that all of your ties and issues be severed and that absolution be granted. Rehash as many times as you need to, depending on the situation, to make sure all ties are made!

Kinship:

Use a moonstone and rose quartz mix for kinship issues. Wear them or carry them with you, and be available to anyone who appears in your life, as you will attract your own companions.

Dissatisfaction:

Use moss agate to ground yourself and let go of disappointments in your life, as it has a calming and releasing energy. Hold this between your two hands outside and stand shoeless in the grass. Close your eyes and inhale deeply to unwind. Appreciate the entirety of the sounds and energy you are getting for 15 minutes!

Nerve BLADDER:

Place one hematite in your lower back and one at your feet while lying on your stomach. Next, place two Clear Quartz crystals, one on each side of your midriff, and unwind for 15 minutes to help ease nerve and bladder issues.

Sex CONFUSION:

Carry or wear a Golden Enhydro Herkimer, no matter how much you might expect it to help with sexual confusion.

GENERAL HEALING:

Turquoise is an incredible general healer. You can wear or convey this when you need additional recovery energy. In the same way, if you rest for 15 minutes surrounded by turquoise, healing energy will flow through your body and make you feel energized.

Liberality:

Generosity starts at home with some jade. Heft this around in your pocket for at least seven days for the fullest effect. You can likewise make a Jade Pearl solution, charge it for six hours, and gently fog all spaces of your home once a day for seven days.

Gum disease:

Make a topaz and clear quartz remedy, charge for three minutes, and wash orally with the charged water multiple times every day.

GLAUCOMA:

For 15 minutes, lie down and place a Tanzine Aura Quartz crystal over each eye and a Clear Quartz crystal over your third eye chakra, pointing upwards.

GOOD FORTUNE:

Carry Bloodstone for 5 days and watch the favorable luck begin coming your way!

Appreciation:

Cobalt turns out to be extraordinary for appreciation issues! Wear it as a wristband or carry it in your pockets on your dominant side for the best outcomes.

Melancholy:

During times of adversity, keep Apache Tears in your pocket. You can likewise rest with them and encompass your actual body with them for a more powerful meeting.

Establishing:

To assist with establishing issues, wear black tourmaline as an anklet. Wear this for at least 6 hours per day and feel the energy being directed into Mother Earth to help you establish completely! For best outcomes, wear an anklet on every lower leg!

Gathering WORK:

While working on group work meetings, place two White Spirit Quartz stones in opposite corners of the room.

Divine messenger CONNECTION:

Even if you're just taking a break and relaxing during your reflection meetings, put Petalite all around you. Make sure to focus on signs that begin to seem more grounded in your life!

Blame:

Carry or wear a leopardskin jasper and a rose quartz blend for seven days to ease feelings of blame. Make sure to purify altogether a short time later.

GUMS:

For sore gums, put mahogany obsidian in a small bowl of water and let it sit for 15 minutes. Eliminate the crystal and tenderly rub the charged water over the spaces that are messing you up. You can likewise use this as an oral flush.

Propensity BREAKING ISSUES:

You can wear or carry golden obsidian, as well as encircle yourself with it, depending on your preference! The best way to spread this vibrational energy is to make a Golden Obsidian Jewel Remedy, charge it for 60 minutes, and frequently moisten all the places you are in. You can also place golden obsidian on all sides of the room where you spend the most time!

Hair Growth:

Make a Snowflake Obsidian diamond mixture, charge it for 2 hours, and wash your hair with this charged water or simply wet your hair down when required.

Visualizations:

Lying down for 20 minutes, place an ocean jasper over each eye and hematite at the bottom of your feet. Make sure to purge when finished.

Hand Pain:

Make a carnelian and clear quartz pearl mixture and charge for 2 hours. Delicately fog your hands or absorb them with this charged water.

Bliss:

Malachite and Rose Quartz joined the guests in a happy vibration! Wear these together on a chain or pendant as near your heart chakra as could be expected!

Agreement:

Milky Quartz is an extraordinary vibrational hotspot for amicable sentiments. Place one in each room of your home and purify it once a week!

Roughage FEVER:

Wear citrine in a pendant as much as possible to alleviate hay fever symptoms. You can also use citrine to make a diamond mixture, charge it for three minutes, and lightly fog your whole body.

Migraines:

For cerebral pain, take three amethyst crystals and rest. Spot one on each side of your head and one at your crown chakra, all pointing upwards. Rest and unwind while your cerebral pain disappears!

Solid HAIR:

For shinier and better hair, make a pearl mixture of mica, charge it for three minutes, and wash your hair or wet your hair down with this charged water.

HEARING:

Agate and rhodonite can help with hearing problems. When you're resting, put one on each side of your head and let the vibrational healing energies do their job. You can also put them under your pillow while sleeping to absorb the energies at night!

HEART:

Lie down and place bloodstone and rose quartz over your heart chakra for 15 minutes to ease heart issues.

Acid reflux:

Lie down and place one clear quartz crystal on each side of your chest and one at your crown chakra, pointing upwards. Next, place a rose quartz over your heart chakra and a citrine over your sun-oriented plexus chakra. Unwind for 15-minute time spans.

Warmth RASH:

Make a fluorite and amethyst pearl remedy with cool spring water charged for three minutes, and tenderly fog the territories that are affected.

Wonderful Energies:

Place celestite around you when you're meditating or having fun, or at the very least, put it under your pillow to improve your connections with like-minded people.

HEEL SPURS:

To relieve pain and manifestations, lie down on your stomach and place a hematite over the heel spike and a carnelian on the back of your knee for 15 minutes, three times a day.

HEMORRHOIDS:

Carry bloodstones in your pockets to help relieve the pain and irritation caused by hemorrhoids.

HERPES:

For flare-ups, rest and place fluorite on the opposing sides of your lower hip district and a clear quartz crystal above your navel. Unwind and inhale gradually. This vibrational recovery should be done once every day for three continuous days.

Hiccups:

Make an amethyst and lapis lazuli pearl remedy, charge for 5 minutes, and wash with the charged water for hiccups. Relive each moment until the hiccups stop.

Privacy Issues:

When working with contemplation or healing gatherings, surround the individual with two apache-tear gemstones and have them hold one in each hand.

Positive Attitude:

Elestial Quartz and Herkimer Jewels can be used as a shield while you think things over and can be traded in for a meeting that will make you feel better.

Urticaria:

Lay down and put clear quartz crystals around your body so that they all point clockwise. Hold an amber piece in addition to one of the hives. Turn this counter-clockwise several times before moving on to the next hive region until all of them have been chipped away at with these healing vibrations.

Home Protection:

Ensure that each room in your home contains one piece of clear quartz and one piece of black obsidian. Place them in the opposite corners of each room after cleaning them and charging them for insurance. Be certain to clean them every month!

Genuineness:

If you wear or carry Amazonite for five days, you will notice a shift in your behavior, feelings, and thoughts regarding trust issues.

Expectation:

Carry a combination of Amazonite and Aqua Aura to help with expectation concerns. This is best accomplished over several days. When you're done, try to cleanse.

Hormonal Changes:

Green fluorite can be used to help with hormonal disorders, especially in women. To help keep these changes in balance, put this crystal in a whole shower bottle for two hours and fog yourself from head to toe once a day. Avoid using moonstone because it will aggravate hormonal fluctuations!

Aggression:

Carry or wear Ajoite on your body, not in a satchel, to help relieve tension, stress, and all the bad feelings that come with it.

House Clearing:

Use marcasite at your home clearing meeting to improve the energy and capacity of the work that is being done. You can also use the crystal vibration switch stick before streaming your home.

Kind Energy:

Wear apatite around your throat chakra to draw in more beneficial energy. Quietude Kunzite can help you keep it in your emanation fields for 20 minutes every day! You can rest with it or contemplate. Keep your choices open!

Humor:

To see more humor in everyday life and situations, carry around some fluorite that has been changed for this purpose for a week.

Yearning:

Wear an apatite necklace around your neck to help battle hunger issues while fasting.

Hyper:

Wear hematite around your left lower leg to quiet hyperenergy.

Extreme touchiness:

Combining aventurine and rose quartz for touchiness is awesome! The mix mends and solace simultaneously. Wear or carry these crystals for three days to feel their full effects.

Mania:

Place Marcasite in the spaces that are tricky, just as you would heft this around with you in your energy fields to quiet panic issues.

Vision Idealism:

Bloodstone can chip it away! This is a simple cycle: focus on your goal while holding this in your dominant hand for 15 minutes every day for five days. If you have extra time, please keep this with you or in the space where you spend the majority of your energy!

Brightening Healing:

Use a Shaman Phantom Quartz during a light healing meeting to improve the meeting's capacity and strength.

Creative mind:

Rest and unwind with Clear Calcite for 20 minutes, and then start your meeting to generate new ideas. Get the pencil, drawing cushion, PC, project, or whatever it is you are dealing with. Keep your clear calcite on hand during this opportunity to keep your creative juices flowing.

Safe System:

Wearing a blue quartz necklace with a copper case and chain will help your immune system and keep you safe.

Restlessness:

Carry a mix of amethyst and blue lace agate with you for at least seven days, and your understanding of even the littlest irritations will improve.

Acid reflux:

Sit in a comfortable chair with your feet flat on the floor. For 10 minutes, hold a citrine crystal over your sacral chakra and a clear quartz crystal over your sun-based plexus chakra with your dominant hand. Unwind and scrub the crystals after each use.

Irritation:

For aggravation issues, use a blue lace agate to help mitigate these manifestations. Hold this irritated area and turn the crystal counterclockwise to pull out the stuck, bad energy that is causing the irritation. Do this for 10 minutes two times per day until the space is leveled out!

Impacting Issues:

When dealing with upsetting situations, use a rose quartz to calm down and bring balance. Carry this on your body at these times!

Internal Alignment:

By surrounding yourself with crystals or holding an old piece of quartz in your dominant hand during reflection meetings, you can feel more rooted.

Internal Identity Issues:

To help the effectiveness of an Inner Child healing meeting, get your rhodochrosite and center your intention before you start your meeting. Keep this with you during your energy, healing, or treatment meetings for more effective advancement.

Inward Ear:

Lie down with four Rhodonite stones and spot one on your throat chakra, one on each side of your head at ear level, and then keep going with one on your third eye chakra. Rest and unwind for 20 minutes all at once to help settle issues with the inward ear.

Inward Peace:

Try using chrysocolla because it calms and soothes the heart chakra and is thought to help with problems of world peace. Wear it in a copper encasement on a long chain around your neck, as close to your heart chakra as possible.

Bug Bites:

Use citrine and clear quartz pearls as a cure for tingling, stinging, and eating bugs. Charge the mixture for an hour, then, as required, lightly fog the affected areas. Let the air dry for the best outcomes.

Bugs:

Make an angelite diamond mixture, charge it for three minutes, and delicately fog the entirety of the spaces that the creepy crawlies are disturbing, like plants or even in your home or office.

Frailty:

For weakness, wear rhodochrosite around your neck, as close to your heart chakra as possible. You can also use a shower with rhodochrosite to help with these issues in your quality fields.

Understanding Into Self:

Wear a Tiger's Eye accessory, wristband, or anklet for knowledge of your actual self. Begin to notice appropriate responses seemingly appearing out of nowhere! For best outcomes, wear each of the three!

Sleeping disorder:

If you have trouble falling or staying asleep, put an amethyst under your pillow before bed and make sure it is facing up. If you thrash around a great deal in your sleep, you can make a crystal pocket and sew this into a pillowcase, or even spot this under your bed where your head would be in an arrangement. Again, ensure it is facing upwards, and don't allow the pets to get to it!

Motivation:

Carry tourmaline with the rest of your personal effects, or spot it in the space where you invest the greater part of your energy searching for motivation!

Senses:

Wear lapis lazuli on your predominant hand or wrist and one on your contralateral lower leg to draw upon your very own impulses and trust in them more.

Intelligence:

Combine jade, rose quartz, and lapis lazuli for the best outcomes when searching for a scholarly lift. Carry them in your pocket at all times. You can also encircle yourself with them while sleeping to give yourself an extra boost!

INTERCONNECTEDNESS:

Carry or wear a blend of yellow and orange jade, customized for interconnection, for seven days. Make sure to scrub subsequently.

Proximity:

For proximity issues, ensure you wear lavender jade or have this set in every one of the four corners of the room you are in for the best outcomes.

Instinct:

Turn to a blend of moss agate and malachite for boosting your instinct. When they work together, they help the two sides of your cerebrum and your actual cognition find balance. You can put them in your pocket or put them all around your body and meditate with them.

Natural Dream:

Place an amethyst and jade stone together under your pad before bed. It is ideal on the off chance that you put them in a crystal pocket and secure this to your pad. This combination creates brilliant vibrational energy for having instinctive dreams!

Bigotry:

Use rhodonite when managing the narrow-mindedness of companions, family, and even outsiders. This is an awesome stone to have convenient in your pocket or tote, as no one can really tell when these issues will spring up!

Thoughtfulness:

Try meditating with a circle of black obsidian around your body to help you think about things.

Touchy Bowl:

Lie down and place halite on one or the other side of your hip territory and hematite over your lower mid-region for 15 minutes all at once.

Jaw Pain:

Use two different crystals, fluorite and rose quartz, to mix for jaw torment. Hold the fluorite first and work in a clockwise motion, turning the stunning from one end to the other. Repeat with rose quartz. Shift back and forth between the two crystals multiple times each. To relieve discomfort, make a diamond remedy, charge it for 2 hours, and gently rub the charged water over the external jawbone.

Desire:

Carry or wear eudialyte to help the green-peered beast.

Stream Lag:

Marascite is effective when encountering plane slack. For 60 minutes of absorption, wear this as a pendant or chain around your neck.

Joint Pain:

Apply azurite to the painful joint for 15 minutes at a time to ease the pain. For many joint pains, put water in a shower bottle and let it sit for 20 minutes. Then, lightly mist the area and let it air dry. You can likewise use this charged water by adding a couple of drops to any cream or balm you may use.

Venturing meetings:

To improve your venture meetings, travel while surrounded by rotating crystals of Indicolite quartz and hematite.

Equity/LEGAL MATTERS:

Carry or wear Jade with you when addressing a legitimate issue!

KARMA HEALING:

Use blue fluorite to improve karma healing sessions or your own personal karma issues. Use this during your contemplation sessions by holding it in your dominant hand or encircling yourself with it. Make sure to scrub the crystal subsequently!

KARMIC MATRIX HEALING:

Use rutile quartz during your Karmic Matrix Healing meeting for more effective outcomes.

Kidney Issues:

Use smoky quartz and yellow topaz to help with kidney problems. Lie on your stomach, have a yellow topaz placed over your solar plexus chakra, and two smoky quartz stones placed on either side of your kidney region to help with the side effects.

Graciousness Mindset:

Observe how your mindset changes over the course of seven days while wearing chrysoprase as a pendant for a definitive result.

KUNDALINI ENERGY:

Use ammonite in contemplation meetings to enhance your Kundalini energy. You can also use this at your recovery or energy meetings. Just make sure to hold it in your dominant hand.

Laryngitis:

Make a Clear Quartz, Lapis Lazuli, and Smoky Quartz jewel remedy and charge it for 60 minutes. On a case-by-case basis, swish with the charged water as frequently as possible. After you wash, rest and spot the Clear Quartz over your third eye chakra facing upward, the Lapis Lazuli over your throat chakra, and the Smoky Quartz over your sun-based plexus chakra for 15 minutes to acquire extra vibrational recovery.

Initiative:

Carry or wear Blue Topaz with you for 6 hours every day for 5 days, and your disposition shift will increase trust in your administration capacities.

LEG CRAMPS:

Place the hematite over the affected area and turn it first in a clockwise direction and then in the opposite direction, going back and forth between the two until the pinching stops.

Torpidity:

Carry, wear, or spot an Orange Drusy Quartz under a pad while resting to battle dormant issues.

Giving up:

Pick up a clear quartz stone and hold it with two hands. Zero in on the issue you want to relinquish. Direct the entirety of the considerations, energy, and feelings into this quartz and let the quartz take them on. Head outside and cover your quarts in a space that won't be upset for seven days. Make sure to check where you covered it! Let the quartz and Mother Earth fix these energies and issues you have given them. Make sure to uncover the quartz after seven days and purify it completely!

LICE:

Make a hematite and clear quartz diamond mixture, charge for 2 hours, and delicately fog all individuals, spots, and things that could be affected by this issue.

Light Sensitivity:

Rhodonite can help you fight the effects of light. Wear one on your dominant hand or wrist and another on your opposing lower leg.

Life Overview:

For a meeting to discuss your daily life plan, surround your body with celestite. You ought to have at least eight crystals framing a circle. More can be added if you want to expand the energy yield.

Listening Skills:

To improve your listening skills, keep Cerussite with you for seven days straight.

Liver:

Use aquamarine and yellow topaz together for liver issues. Lay on your stomach, and have someone put the two crystals over your sun-oriented plexus chakra for 15 minutes while you relax. Make sure to purify the crystals when you are finished with your meeting. Depending on the situation, repeat as often as possible.

LIVER SPOTS:

Make a yellow topaz and citrine pearl remedy, charge for 60 minutes, and delicately fog all liver spots multiple times every day for the best outcomes.

Depression:

Carry or wear cobaltite to combat depression. If this is a problem you're having at home, put it in the two opposite corners of your main living area as well. Purge consistently.

LONG LIFE:

If you want to live longer and longer, you should carry or wear moonstone as much as you can, especially during the full moon. You can likewise put one moonstone in each room of your home and office. Make sure to purify them consistently.

LOST OBJECTS:

Charge an infinite fee to track down your lost articles. Hold this in your dominant hand and focus on just the item you are looking for. Try not to allow your brain to meander. Follow your instinct when searching for the lost item.

LOTTO LUCK/GAMBLING:

When playing lottery sorts of games, try to have your

LOVE (PLATONIC):

Wear rhodonite as close as possible to your heart chakra for seven days at a time. Make sure to scrub after every seven-day time frame.

LOVE (ROMANTIC):

Place Sardonyx in the corner of your room, nearest to your bed, and in a kitchen corner, nearest to the oven, and watch how the progressions begin to show in practically no time!

LOVE (UNCONDITIONAL):

Hold one jade and one rose quartz in your hands and center them with the entirety of your aim at the current issue. For the next five days, carry or wear these stones however much is reasonable to anticipate. After five days, you should clean the crystals and accuse them of this plan again. Rehash as frequently as necessary depending on the situation in different spaces of adoration!

Faithfulness:

Issues of dedication can be settled by the vibrational degrees of kyanite. Before carrying or wearing this stone on your actual body, make sure to clean it thoroughly. Changes will begin to show in a couple of days! If you have issues with another person's dependability, place this in your home or office and see the progression show up with the individual inside a couple of days!

Clear Dreaming:

Include your albite in your quality fields if you're using transparent dream meetings, carrying or wearing it to help you see things more clearly during the session.

Karma:

Changing your karma can be done by wearing a solitary pointed Smoky Quartz pendant facing upward! In addition, this crystal can be soaked in water for twenty minutes in a shower container before being used to gently fog a body part or area.

Lungs:

Lie down and place one Indicolite Quartz on each side of your body, close to your lungs. Next, place a clear quartz crystal at your heart chakra, facing upward, and inhale deeply for 15 minutes.

Lupus:

To help ease Lupus indications, carry a mixture of hematite, clear quartz, and rhodonite in your pocket, purse, or pendant.

Making New Patterns:

Make a purple rainbow fluorite diamond solution, charge for three hours, and tenderly fog the spaces of your home or office. Rehash at regular intervals while energy designs shift.

Male Energetic Balance:

Make a green tourmaline diamond solution, charge it for 2 hours, and fog your whole home or office with this delicately, particularly in the corners!

Showing:

Hold smoky quartz and citrine in your dominant hand while concentrating on your appearance for 15 minutes. Ensure that you carry them with you for the next few days and track the development of your cravings.

Marriage Issues:

For a more connected marriage, have the spouse scrub, charge, and program an aquamarine. Request that your companion do the same for a rose quartz. At that point, the two of them switch and carry the contrary crystal with them for seven days. Depending on the circumstances, rehash in order to strengthen the relationship.

Development:

Carry or wear malachite with you to achieve a more developed demeanor at work, home, and when seeing someone.

MEASLES:

To help ease measles manifestations, make a diamond solution of carnelian and hematite, charge for 60 minutes, and delicately fog the individual from head to toe three times each day!

Reflection:

Before you start your contemplation session, put amethyst and clear quartz crystals around you. This will make it feel more special. Make sure that most of them are pointing inward, and clean them regularly.

Recollections:

To let go of old, painful memories, hold a rose quartz in each hand and put a piece of hematite at your feet while you're relaxed or thinking. Zero in on the memory and let go of the entirety of the sentiments and feelings that rise to the surface.

Menopause:

Carry the Black Onyx and Howlite blend in your pocket or pouch to help relieve menopausal symptoms!

Mental Attachment:

Lay down and place a yellow phantom quartz on each side of your head, followed by a fluorite at your third eye chakra. Unwind and rest for 15 minutes.

Intellectual ability:

Meditate or lay down with an opal to expand your intellectual knowledge. This will take advantage of a more significant amount of your cerebrum's capacity each time you use it.

Mental Cleanser:

Lapis lazuli should be able to cleanse the mind. Rest on your back and spot one on each side of your head and one at your crown chakra. Unwind and inhale profoundly and gradually for 15 minutes. You can also hold a lapis lazuli in your dominant hand while sitting in a chair and gradually work with the energy of the crystal, moving it clockwise around your head, third eye, and crown chakras. Make sure to purge the crystals a short time later!

Meridian and Marmas Cleaning:

Use a lodestone in your meridian, and marmas are cleansing gatherings that boost the ability to heal and clean.

Digestion:

For better digestion, put Amazonite in your bathwater and take a warm, wet shower before you start your day.

Headache:

Lie down and place one Tanzine Aura Quartz on each side of your throat, one over your third eye chakra, and a Clear Quartz over your crown chakra. Relax for 15 minutes, then rehash based on the situation.

MIRROR ENERGY:

Mirror energy is the point at which you take on someone else's mindset or feelings. This can be settled by using hematite. Keep this in your pocket or purse for best results, as no one knows when this will happen. Hematite will help in diverting, rather than engaging, these energies.

Setback:

To fix problems in your life, take out your black tourmaline and slowly work on your emanation fields, drawing out all negative and stale energy.

Cash:

Carrying a piece of pyrite in your wallet, tote, or checkbook is all it takes to attract more money into your life.

Emotional episodes:

During common emotional episodes, use Jet to regain equilibrium and balance your emotions and temperament. Sit with your feet flat on the ground and grasp this with both hands. Consider all of the emotions and sentiments that have been fluctuating and changing in your life right now. Feel all of them as though they were changing at that moment. Immediately release the Jet to the floor by opening your hands. Inhale and exhale a full breath. Rise to your feet and thoroughly purge the jet!

MOON ENERGY:

Wear a moonstone around your lower leg every other day, during, and after each new and full moon to raise your vibrational association with the moon's energy.

Movement Sickness:

During times of movement infection, keep aquamarine in your pocket or hold it in your dominant hand. This will help you feel better.

Inspiration:

For more inspiration, make a point to put carnelian where you invest most of your energy, regardless of whether you are busy working or at home, to give you that extra persuasive lift.

Engine SKILLS:

To improve the performance of your engine, carry or wear quartz with mica for a week straight. Make sure to cleanse for the next seven days.

MOUTH:

Use a blend of lapis lazuli and rose quartz for mouth issues. Rest, spot the Lapis Lazuli over your throat chakra, place a Rose Quartz crystal on each side of your mouth, and unwind for 10 minutes at a time.

Muscle spasms:

Make a treatment with an Amazonite Jewel, let it sit for three minutes, and then gently fog the muscles twice a day. You can likewise use this water and add a couple of drops to any cream or balm you are using. For an immediate goal, place this crystal inside two circles of the affected territory and go clockwise to draw out the negative energies.

Legends:

Wear rainforest jasper around the two lower legs to help manage fantasies being spread about you or your way of life.

Nail Growth:

Use obsidian to assist nails in developing further, longer, and faster. Delicately rub the nails with this crystal three times each day. Similarly, you can make charged water and place a couple of drops on each pin three times per day for faster results.

Sickness:

Lie down and place topaz over your stomach region and one clear quartz crystal on each side of your mid-region. Inhale gradually and profoundly for 10 minutes.

NECK STRAIN:

Start by holding the chrysoprase in your dominant hand and slowly moving it around your neck. Next, hang the crystal preposterously clockwise. On the other hand, take the crystal in your dominant hand and turn it around your entire channel. Last, pivot the crystal counter-clockwise, preposterous.

Cynicism:

To address negative vibrations, take a stab at using black and green tourmaline. You can put these in one corner of every room in your home, vehicle, or office. Make sure to scrub them two times per month.

Disregard:

 Hematite and rose quartz can help you deal with feelings of being ignored if you wear them as a pendant.

Apprehension:

You can wear turquoise as a beautiful piece of jewelry, and no one will know it helps you with this problem. Jewelry works best for this condition because it is tailored to your specific body.

Sensory system:

Wearing amber and black tourmaline together in a pendant can help you get better if you're having problems with your senses.

Fresh start:

When you want a fresh start, make a moonstone pearl remedy. Permit it to charge for three hours and delicately fog all regions and issues that need a fresh start. It is ideal to do it at the hour of a new moon.

NEW SURROUNDINGS:

Place brown jade in each room of your new home or at your office to assist you with changing the unique environmental factors and energy vibrations.

Bad dreams:

Sleep with a mix of amethyst and fluorite under your pillow to manage bad dreams.

NIGHT SWEATS:

Sleep with Indicolite quartz under your pillow to help ease night sweats.

NOSE:

Lie down and place a fluorite over your nose and a clear quartz crystal underneath your nose, and unwind for 10 minutes to help ease indications.

NOSE BLEED:

Place sapphire or carnelian over the extension of the nose during a nosebleed to stop the bleeding.

Seeing CHAKRA ALIGNMENT:

Place a black onyx stone on each chakra territory, beginning with your root chakra and moving gradually up through your crown chakra.

Deafness:

Place hematite and petrified wood around the numb area and swap stones in a circle of growth. Rest and inhale profoundly, unwinding for 15 minutes all at once. Purify them after every brief span.

Sustaining:

To improve a supporting side, work with a moonstone. Spot this in a space you use the most or in various areas of your home, just as you wear or convey this on your actual body.

OBJECTIVITY:

Place Rainforest Jasper in two opposite corners of your home or office where you can spend more energy to help with this problem.

Fanatical ISSUES:

Carry or wear a White Spirit Quartz to control the top issues.

Open the Mind:

Lie down and place aragonite over your third eye chakra for 20 minutes per day to open your brain to additional astounding prospects each time you do this.

Receptiveness:

To turn out to be more open to thoughts, individuals, and circumstances, convey or wear Astrophyllite for seven days straight. Make sure to scrub subsequently.

Positive thinking:

Wanting to turn out more idealistic? Wear Chalcedony around your neck for the best results!

Hierarchical ABILITIES:

Organizing isn't for everyone, but you can use Jasper to increase your authority! Spot this in the two inverse corners of your office or home, where you do the most getting organized, and your abilities will soar.

OUT-OF-BODY EXPERIENCE (OBE):

Use apophyllite when working with out-of-body encounters during your meeting to improve the experience and associations.

OVERREACTION ISSUES:

If you are one of the individuals who tends to overreact to circumstances when all is said and done, have a go at hauling a moonstone around with you as a feature of your general everyday schedule. A moonstone will help quiet your enthusiastic responses!

OVER-STIMULATION:

Lay down and put a piece of blue quartz over your heart chakra. Then, take deep breaths for 15 minutes to calm yourself down.

OVER THINKING:

Make a lattice of Howlite in a bit of territory close to where you, for the most part, are overthinking reasoning issues, for example, on a table in your office or at home. Make sure this is close to the areas where you have the most trouble to change the effects.

Torment:

To ease general agony over a physical issue or illness, use a blend of turquoise and rose quartz together. Place them in close proximity to the affected area for five minutes while aimed directly at the area. At that point, gradually turn the crystals clockwise for an additional 2 minutes. This will aid in drawing out the found negative energy and restoring a positive energy flow to alleviate the pain. Continue to shift back and forth between the two until the torment dies down.

Palpitation:

If you have palpitations, hold hematite and rose quartz in your dominant hand over your heart chakra and take slow, deep breaths for 15 minutes.

Pancreas:

Lie on your stomach and look for two emeralds on each side of your midriff, as well as a smokey quartz in your waist. Rest and unwind for 15 minutes. Rehashing depends on the situation.

Fits of anxiety:

Take a green phantom quartz in each hand and place it on the ground. Close your eyes, put your hands loosely in your lap, and take deep, slow breaths for 15 minutes to calm an alarm attack.

Distrustfulness:

Wear a mix of hematite and sugilite to battle issues of neurosis.

Interest:

If you are having trouble with support, place four Clear Quartz Crystal Clusters, one on each edge of the room where you spend the most time. Make sure to purify them two times every month!

Enthusiasm:

Make sure to wear garnet for individuals and circumstances requiring loads of energy!

Aloof ENERGY ISSUES:

Wear blue jade around your correct lower leg for five days straight for detached energy issues.

Previous existence Healing:

Utilize Tanzanite during a previous existence healing meeting to improve the work being completed.

Previous existence RECALL:

Use Amber to review your previous existence, recollections, and issues. To improve the effectiveness of a last-minute existence or reflection meeting, encircle yourself with this.

Tolerance:

Patience issues can be settled with rhodonite. They help educate and raise the vibrational level of your quiet conduct. Mix them into a solution, let the water base sit for an hour, and then lightly fog the area you want to treat or the person from head to toe.

Harmony:

Make a jewel remedy of rose quartz and blue tourmaline for the best outcomes. Charge the water base for an hour, and then use fog to restore balance anywhere you need to. On the off chance that you need a more tranquil home and living climate, fog every space of your home.

Genuine feelings of serenity:

Wear a sapphire pendant to gain significant serenity during battle seasons.

Discernment:

Carry a desert rose around in your pocket to build your view of thoughts, spots, individuals, and circumstances.

Individual POWER:

Wear a mix of garnet and emerald for two days around your heart chakra to improve your own force.

Cynical BEHAVIOR:

Wear or carry a Hawk's Eye to aid in combating critical behavior. If the behavior is going on in a space like the office, place two of them there, one in each opposite corner of the room.

Fears:

Carry a Blue Opal in your pocket or tote to manage fears that emerge. At the point when they turn their heads, haul this out and tenderly hold it close to your heart chakra and inhale profoundly.

PLANT ENERGY:

Wear a moss agate around your lower leg to connect to plant energies!

PLANT GROWTH:

Put cerrussite in your plants that have been pruned or put this stone around them to keep bugs away and help the roots grow. Make a diamond solution, charge for 60 minutes, and water the plant with this mixture depending on the situation.

Toxin IVY RASH:

If you come into contact with the toxic substance, you will begin to break out in an irritating rash. Make a diamond mixture of black tourmaline and aventurine and charge for three minutes. Depending on the situation, gently fog this everywhere on your actual body from head to toe as frequently as possible!

Inspiration:

Wear or carry a poppy jasper to feel happy, full of energy, and in a good mood all day.

Post-pregnancy Issues:

For the best results, wear a rhodonite pendant and a black onyx anklet to combat blue eyes.

Force Animal Communication:

Utilize a mixture of Shaman Phantom Quartz and Dalmatian Stone during power creature communication gatherings to strengthen the bond.

Common sense:

Are you having reasonableness issues? Wear a single Tiger's Eye to your left lower leg or wrist for three days, and you'll notice a difference!

Untimely AGING:

Make a turquoise diamond remedy, charge for 60 minutes, and sprinkle tenderly ludicrous that you require to combat maturing signs.

PRESENT ENERGY:

Need assistance remaining at the current time and place? Carry a Staurolite, also known as a Fairy Cross, with you as much as possible in your pocket!

Dangerous ISSUES:

Make a Red Jasper diamond remedy, charge for 60 minutes, and tenderly fog all spaces of your home or office to uncover hazardous issues before they become a significant issue. This is to bring the hidden problems you may not have thought about yet out sooner, so you can chip away at them before they get crazy.

Extending ENERGY:

Use yellow jasper to extend energy during healing meetings. Before you begin, make sure this is in your dominant hand and that you are very grounded. This helps when working on specific healing sessions and making more grounded, enthusiastic associations.

Prescience Prophecy capacities:

Encircle yourself with this during reflections, while diverting, or wear it as near your third eye chakra as could be expected. While resting, place the emerald over your third eye chakra and start to ponder.

Flourishing:

Carry an ammonite in your pocket, purse, or wallet to get improved success vibrations.

Insurance:

Onyx and black tourmaline are excellent for security issues. They help ground and repel negative energy. Best ideas, wear one as a pendant and one as an ankle. This will ensure the repulse of every lousy point and issue.

Clairvoyant ATTACK:

To forestall and ward off mystic assaults, a conveyor wears Aqua Aura. Use this in the mix with assurance crystals, too!

Clairvoyant DEVELOPMENT:

Lapis lazuli, amethyst, and clear quartz crystals are an effective blend for upgrading mystic events. Rest on your back and spot the lapis lazuli over your throat chakra, the amethyst over your third eye chakra, and the clear quartz over your crown chakra. During this period, center your expectations and ruminate too. You can also carry or wear these crystal blends around with you to constantly bring their abilities into your airways. Also, it's important to surround yourself with crystals and trade them in a circle during regular meditation meetings.

PUBLIC SPEAKING:

Make sure you have hematite and carnelian with you when you talk to help you deal with current problems.

Unadulterated THOUGHT:

Lay down and put azurite over your third eye chakra for 15 minutes to get a clear, deep look into your thoughts and mind.

Cleansing:

Make a Smoky Quartz Jewel remedy, charge it for 2 hours, and delicately fog your actual body gently from head to toe, or for the whole territory too.

Stop SMOKING:

To help you quit smoking, convey or wear a Botswana agate.

Anger:

Carry or wear carnelian with you to combat feelings of aggression. For best outcomes, wear or convey this on your dominant side.

RAINBOW ENERGY:

Consider incorporating rainbow fluorite into your meetings in order to enhance a rainbow energy association.

Fast CHANGE:

To achieve a quick change, make a moldavite and clear quartz mixture and delicately fog all spaces in your home or office. Next, place the moldavite and clear quartz in the far corners of your home to help increase the vibrational energy.

RASHES:

Make a red agate jewel mixture, charge it for 60 minutes, and delicately sprinkle the rash region three times each day for the best outcomes.

Soundness:

Sodalite is used for issues of discernment. Bring or wear this stone on these occasions!

RAZOR BUMPS:

Gently rub a rhodonite diamond solution, which has been charged for three minutes, over the razor bumps three times each day!

Acknowledgment ISSUES:

Wear amethyst as close to your heart chakra as possible to help with recognition issues.

Getting Energy:

For accepting energy from an individual or meeting, ensure you have a clear quartz on or in your dominant hand to make the gathering more grounded.

Recovering FROM ILLNESS:

Make sure to have as much aquamarine as possible around the person who is recovering from illness. This will accelerate the way toward healing.

Purge every day.

Recovering FROM SURGERY:

When recovering from a medical procedure, try to place turquoise, aquamarine, and clear quartz crystals near the individual or in the room they invest the most energy in. scrub day by day.

Recovery:

For recovery issues, use an Elestial Quartz jewel solution and charge it for 2 hours. Gently fog the whole body for the best outcomes.

REIKI ENHANCEMENT:

Make it a point to bring a pink crackle quartz to every Reiki meeting to improve the energy. Encircle yourself with this or hold it in your dominant hand when working.

REINTEGRATION:

Use an Eilat Stone for reintegration purposes. Make sure you wear or carry this for five days straight!

Dismissal:

Make a jewel remedy of carnelian and rose quartz for the best outcomes, and charge for 60 minutes. Delicately fog your whole body, from your head to your toes, once every day for these issues, along with any spaces that raise dismissal issues!

Restoration:

Make a Purpurite pearl mixture, charge for 60 minutes, and tenderly fog the zones out of luck.

Delivery THE PAST:

Hold the azurite in your hands and think only about what you want to say about the past. Focus all of your energy on these things and goals, and let the vibrational energies of the azurite stone take hold of them and free you from them. Make sure to purify after each use.

Delivering:

Use a Phantom Quartz crystal for delivering issues by wearing it around your neck for five days.

Connections:

Try using a malachite and rose quartz blend. They will unite joy, love, regard, and delicate quieting energies. Wear or convey them together during these occasions and watch how the connections develop!

Repel Lower Energies:

Make sure you convey Hematite and Smoky Quartz in your pocket when all over town to help repel lower vibrating energies.

Hatred ISSUES:

Malachite on a long chain worn as a pendant during times of disdain can help with these problems.

Anxious:

Take a steaming shower—no sweat—for your fretfulness issues.

A tendency to fidget When hitting the hay before a battle, wear Falcon's Eye around your lower legs to keep you from fidgeting.

Renewal:

Make a mixture of carnelian, citrine, and clear quartz pearl, charge for 2 hours, and gently fog the area, individual, or person in need of assistance.

Stiffness:

Combine amber and carnelian to ease ailments. Use a water base for these two or three minutes and delicately fog the affected zones!

ROOM CLEANSING:

Make an amber pearl mixture, charge for 60 minutes, and delicately fog all room spaces from roof to floor, including furniture, corners, and anything in the room except electrical gadgets.

ROSACEA:

Make a jewel remedy with amethyst and citrine, let it sit for an hour, and then fog all the affected areas three times a day.

Trouble:

Wear an Indicolite quartz and a rose quartz pendant near your heart chakra for seven days. Make sure to purge thoroughly.

SCABS:

Make a jewel remedy with carnelian and cobaltite, charge it for 2 hours, and delicately pat or fog the region that is affected.

Shortage:

Mix emerald and hematite and put it around yourself or your area to fight feelings of lack.

SCARS:

Make a Cobalite diamond mixture, charge it for 60 minutes, and delicately pat the charged water over the scars. Depending on the situation, repeat as often as possible.

Dispersed ENERGY:

Wear hematite on your lower leg to help manage dissipated energy. For an additional lift, wear one on your other wrist too!

Foretelling:

Use celestite groups to improve your Foretelling abilities and meetings. Ensure the entirety of the focus is facing upwards during your meeting.

Occasional AFFECTIVE DISORDER:

During SAD, make sure to wear the septarian. Make sure to scrub this at regular intervals.

SECURITY:

Make a tree agate pearl solution, charge it for 60 minutes, and delicately fog the regions or individuals managing security issues. Rehash as frequently as necessary.

SELF CARE:

Carry or wear Epidote as often as you can to get gentle reminders to take care of your body, such as getting enough rest, eating well, and exercising to keep a healthier body.

Poise:

Wear or convey Gray Hawk's Eye with you when you feel wild!

Confidence ISSUES:

Carry or wear Chalcopyrite for seven days straight to help you manage confidence issues.

Pointless ISSUES:

A mix of smoky quartz and citrine can help you chip away at silly problems. Convey or wear these two together for the greatest advantage!

SELF HEALING:

Amber is a brilliant method to support anyone's self-healing! Spot this territory for 20 minutes. On the off chance that you're chipping away at general self-healing, surround yourself with this before your meeting starts.

Confidence:

Try wearing a rose quartz pendant as close as possible to your heart chakra to chip away at issues of self-esteem. You can also support this vibrational energy of self-esteem by soaking in a bath filled with water for 20 minutes and then washing up!

Dignity:

Wear a mix of rainforest jasper and rose quartz together for seven days to help support your sense of pride.

Narrow-mindedness ISSUES:

Hold Howlite close to your heart chakra once per day for seven days and concentrate on being less self-centered, angry, and essential.

Communicating Consciously:

Surround yourself with moldavite while attempting correspondence with whales, dolphins, or others. If you can't contemplate encircling yourself with this, wear it as close to your throat chakra as possible for the best results.

Quietness:

Make an amethyst-jewel solution, charge it for three minutes, and gently fog the territory you are in. Eliminate the amethyst and spot this on the side of a similar room.

SEXUAL IMPROVEMENT:

Place a red jasper in each of the four corners of your room and a smoky quartz under your bed for sexual improvement.

SHAMAN JOURNEY:

Mochi Balls placed in a circle around you during a shamanic excursion will improve your relationship and excursion voyaging!

Shielding Energy:

Place a lapis lazuli and a clear quartz in one corner of each room that needs energy protection. Make sure to scrub twice a month.

Stun ISSUES:

When someone is stunned, it usually results in a massive hit to the energy fields. Rest and spot hematite at your feet chakra, carnelian over your navel, turquoise over your throat chakra, and clear quartz over your crown chakra and at both hand chakras. Rest and unwind for three minutes.

SHOULDER STRAIN:

If you have a shoulder strain or injury, putting chrysoprase within two inches of the area can help. Turn this clockwise to eliminate the negative energy.

Bashfulness:

If you are extremely modest and need to go out and about, convey or wear lepidolite. Even the strongest energies can give this a break for a few days, so try not to rush it.

Effortlessness:

Make a Larimar jewel solution, charge it for three minutes, and gently fog the territories that you need to rearrange, just as you would.

SINGING:

Wear rhodonite as a pendant around your neck to enhance your singing abilities!

SINUS ISSUES:

Make an eilat stone pearl remedy and charge for 60 minutes. You can either delicately pat the region needing vibrational crystal healing or make steam from this charged water to breathe in and recuperate from the inside.

SKIN IRRITATIONS/ISSUES:

Make a mixture of turquoise and clear quartz crystal pearls, let it sit for 60 minutes, and then gently fog the parts of the skin that need help.

Children's Sleep Problems:

For issues with bad dreams, the boogieman, and beasts in the wardrobe or under the bed, place charoite under the bed or in the storage room—any place the youngsters are having issues with these feelings of dread. Involving the child in the creation of a monster repellent shower also places the child in charge of exorcising the evil spirits that frighten them. Charge the water for the splash for three minutes, and let your little one rain the entirety of the terrible boogiemen away!

Rest TALKING:

Put a rainbow fluorite under the person's pillow before bed to stop them from being restless.

Rest WALKING:

If the person has trouble falling asleep, have them wear a rainbow moonstone before bed.

Wheezing:

To help with wheezing, place a lapis lazuli in two inverse corners of the bed edge and a clear quartz in the other two inverse corners of the bed edge.

Collectedness:

Wear iolite around your throat chakra as much as possible when attempting to keep your temper and to help reinforce your solidarity and fortitude.

Socialization:

If you want to improve your social skills, keep Garnet in your pocket whenever you have the chance to meet new people.

SORE THROAT:

Make a blue-quartz mixture, charge for 60 minutes, and rinse with the charged water. Repeat as often as necessary, case by case.

Wounds:

Use carnelian to help with mild injuries on your actual body. Spot this inside two creeps of the sore and turn first clockwise and then counterclockwise, rotating to and fro between the two. Make sure to purify altogether a short time later.

SOUL HEALING:

Use a black opal to make a strong connection and help the client or yourself realize their true soul value to its fullest potential.

SOUL PURPOSE:

It is important to carry chiastolite, also known as the "Cross Stone", when seeking one's spirit purpose. This will help with the vibrational energy of this space. You can likewise encircle yourself with four of them during a contemplation meeting while looking for answers.

SOUL RETRIEVAL:

If you want to get the most out of a spirit recovery meeting, use a lepidocrocite quartz crystal.

Accelerate ENERGY FLOW:

You can speed up the flow of energy through your chakras, qualities, and meridians by wearing a tiger's eye around your two lower legs!

Otherworldly Awakening:

Surround yourself with fluorite during your contemplation meetings, just as you would lay down with similar crystals under your pad to construct an association with them. Convey or wear one for seven days and watch your otherworldly stimulating encounters begin!

Profound BLOCK:

Use a Star Ruby when chipping away at your otherworldly pathway to eliminate blockages. These squares can come in any structure along your way, so keep your Star

However, Ruby could reasonably be expected to be with you in an accessory, pocket, or close to you in your home or office.

Otherworldly CLEANSER:

Wear lapis lazuli for seven days in a row to upgrade and cleanse your spirit!

Immediacy:

Have the individual convey an opal on their dominant side for at least two days to increase unconstrained behavior.

Injuries:

Make a Dalmatian Stone Pearl solution, charge for 60 minutes, and drench the hyperextended territory. If you are unable to soak the area, absorb a perfect towel from the charged water and fold it over the area. Then, using the Dalmatian Stone, locate the inside two corners of the injury and work clockwise to eliminate any residual negative energy.

Security:

Wear or convey a faden quartz and amber blend to expand the strength in your life.

Anxiety in front of large audiences:

Make sure you place a Dumortierite in your pocket before going in front of an audience, so you can reach in and hold it regularly for an additional increase in vibrational energy.

STAMMERING:

Wear or carry blue tourmaline near your throat chakra if possible to help with stammering issues!

Tranquility:

Make a Celestite Jewel solution and gently fog all areas that require quiet.

STOMACH ULCERS:

Rest and put an agate over your stomach area and two clear quartz crystals, one on each side of your body, pointing inward. This will help heal stomach ulcers. Relax for 15 minutes, and then rehash the situation.

Tempests:

For energy security during storms, ensure you place agate in each room of your home or wear this on the off chance you are out and about during a storm.

STRENGTH:

When feeling powerless or needing some more strength, wear a red-banded agate around your lower leg for the best outcomes.

STRESS:

Use an amethyst to cut down on feelings of anxiety. You can use them to decorate your home or office, create a charged water fog, wear them, or carry them on your body.

Obstinacy:

Carry a blend of rose quartz and malachite to ease determination issues.

Examining:

Make sure to bring a sodalite to your investigation meetings so that you can think more critically.

Pen:

Place a fluorite two crawls away from the affected eye. Turn this multiple times clockwise. Next, hold a clear quartz inside the two corners of the eye and turn it clockwise numerous times. Shift back and forth between the two stones for 5 minutes, three times per day!

Subliminal:

Use selenite for subliminal issues. Start by holding this and imagining it bringing white light energy down through your crown chakra, into your actual body, and out through your foot chakras. Next, place this over your third eye chakra to store data in your inner mind.

SUN ENERGY:

Wear a sunstone around your lower leg for 24 hours per day for three days to improve your vibrational association with the sun's energy.

Sunburn:

Make a Dumortierite diamond mixture, let it sit for 60 minutes, and then carefully fog all areas that have been burned by the sun.

Backing ISSUES:

Dark citrine is effective for helping with issues. If you can't get help from anyone else, put it where you spend the most time or energy at home or at work. If you are not giving good help to other people, wear or convey this on your actual body!

Smothered PATTERNS:

Use Apache Tears during reflection or recovery meetings, with one set in each hand and one situated at each foot chakra, to uncover stifled examples.

Sweating:

Make a solution of emerald, carnelian, and clear quartz crystal pearls and let it charge for 60 minutes. This will stop you from sweating too much. First, carefully mist your entire body from head to toe. Next, lightly mist the quality layers that are within two feet of your body to fix these problems.

Growing:

Swelling can be reduced by placing Aquamarine in two crevices of the swollen area and turning it clockwise and then counterclockwise.

SWIMMERS EAR:

Lie down and place hematite over your throat chakra, a clear quartz crystal over your crown chakra pointing upwards, and fluorite on each side of your ears. Relax for 20 minutes to aid in the critical factor and torment.

Ability:

Use Bloodstone to help support your ability! Carry or wear this as much as possible when focusing on your ability issues!

Instructing:

Carry or wear citrine for expanded capacity and energy in the educational field.

TEETH:

For sound teeth, charge some water with fluorite for 15 minutes, and flush your mouth and teeth with this charged water!

Precognition:

To improve association and transmission when using your precognitive abilities, hold an angelite crystal against your third eye chakra.

TENDONITIS:

Lie down and encircle yourself with substitute crystals of clear quartz, rose quartz, and black tourmaline. Use these three stones to make a pearl mixture that lasts an hour, and fog the areas that are affected.

Strain:

Put Black Tourmaline two inches from the pressure point on your body and move it back and forth repeatedly. When the pressure is backing off, turn this clockwise to pull out the excess negative and stale energy.

Musings:

To improve your considerations, use Celestite! Either carry it with you wherever you go or place it in your office and home, where you spend the most time!

THROAT INFECTIONS:

Charge some water with aquamarine and swish three times each day to help ease throat diseases.

TMJ:

Lie down and place three hematite stones around your shoulders, one at the base and one on each side. Next, place an amethyst on each side of your ears and one over your third eye chakra. Unwind for 20 minutes all at once.

Resilience:

Carry or wear chrysoprase with you and place it in two opposite corners of your home or office to help with resistance!

TOOTHACHE:

For toothache torment, charge a bowl of water with aquamarine for 20 minutes. Rub the charged water delicately over your teeth and gum line, or flush your mouth with the charged water.

Decipher Higher Thoughts:

Use Cerussite during your reflection meetings by holding it in your dominant hand. Make sure to write down everything after your meeting, and bring your Cerussite with you so that you can bring your thoughts from a higher plane to this one.

Injury:

Combine Aqua Aura and Rose Quartz for the best outcomes in an injury circumstance. Use this on your physical body or surround yourself with it to ward off bad energy!

Voyaging PROTECTION:

Carry or wear blue obsidian during your season of movement for essential voyaging security!

TREE ENERGY:

Use tree agate to ground yourself and connect with tree energies. Hold this in your dominant hand and select your #1 tree. Try to walk barefoot if you can, and give your tree an embrace. Take a seat at the tree's base and appreciate the energy association.

TREE GROWTH:

Place a tree and moss agate around the base of your tree, shifting back and forth between the two to invigorate tree development. Make a diamond remedy, charge for 60 minutes, and water the tree with this mixture, depending on the situation.

TRUST ISSUES:

Trust issues can be managed via conveying hematite. This reflects all adverse matters, so you can zero in on energy that isn't diverting during these occasions!

TRUTH:

Wear or carry Iolite as much as is reasonably expected to be able to achieve truth issues in a random situation. If you are looking for reality in others, make a point to put Iolite in the four corners of the room that you both invest the most energy in.

TWIN FLAMES:

Program a Blue Aragonite to draw in your twin fire while holding it close to your heart chakra. To the extent that is reasonably possible, carry this with you wherever you go.

Awkward FEELINGS:

If you are feeling uncomfortable, go after a clear quartz, a rose quartz, or an amethyst. Hold them near your heart chakra and take a couple of full breaths, letting out the entirety of the awkward sentiments. If you have them all, encircle yourself with them for a fast arrival of this energy!

UNDERSTANDING:

Wear lapis lazuli in a pendant near your heart chakra to assist with getting through issues.

Hidden world:

To strengthen your connection to the hidden world, use Smoky Spirit Quartz crystals in your meditation and leadership sessions. You can also surround yourself with a circle while using Crystal Healing Tips and Techniques.

URINARY TRACT ENERGIES:

For 15 minutes, lie down and place a Tanzine Aura Quartz over your lower midsection, a Carnelian on each side of your actual body, and Hematite at your feet.

Novel PERSONAL ENERGY:

When working with a group, make a labradorite pearl solution, charge it for an hour before using it, and fog the area gently. This will make it easier for each person to bring their own unique energy to the world.

Interesting LIFE PATH:

Carry or wear Amazonite, however much is required to find your one-of-a-kind life path.

Concealed ENTITIES:

Use Prehnite for inconspicuous substances by putting them around your home, in each corner. You can also carry or wear this when you are not at home to help with these issues!

Undesirable:

Place sugilite in two far corners of a similar room in your home or office to get rid of bad energies.

Upper Chakras:

Whenever you open your upper chakras, make sure you are surrounded by purple agate. If you need to do this with your guides and higher self, encircle yourself in contemplation with purple agate.

VARICOSE VEINS:

Make a yellow topaz diamond mixture, charge it for 60 minutes, and gently fog the varicose veins twice a day for seven days.

VIBRATIONAL ENERGY:

Use a petalite to feel vibrational energies more strongly, especially when working with crystals and gemstones. Hold this in your dominant hand when you are healing or working with crystals or other vibrational energies.

Infants' Illness:

Infants who are sick are given apatite near their heart chakra to help them heal faster.

VISION:

Clear calcite helps with growing vision issues. For best results, place this under your cushion, reflect with it encompassing your actual body or rests, and place it in the center of your eyes, just beneath your third eye chakra!

VISION QUESTS:

Surround yourself with a circle of Petalite during your vision-mission meeting for the best outcomes.

Perceptions:

When zeroing in on representations, add selenite to upgrade your latent capacity. Encircle yourself with them for a higher vibrational level!

VOICE STRENGTHENED:

Use carnelian worn around your neck and throat chakra to reinforce your voice!

Moles:

Make a solution of Marcasite and charge for two hours. Depending on the situation, you can either fog the area or gently pat the area with the charged water.

WATER CHARGE:

With your dominant hand, hold a clear quartz-terminated crystal above a glass of water, and slowly turn the crystal clockwise several times to remove poisons.

WATER ENERGY:

For seven days, carry or wear a combination of Aqua Aura and Aquamarine to increase the vibrations of water.

WATER TRAVEL/SAFETY:

For water travel and security, convey or sport aquamarine on your actual body!

WATERY EYES:

Lie down and place iolite over each eye and a clear quartz crystal over your third eye, facing upward for 10 minutes. Rehash on a case-by-case basis.

WEIGHT GAIN:

To gain weight, use your amber and charge your food 10 minutes before eating to raise the vibrational level.

Weight loss:

Use a blend of moonstone and rose quartz for weight reduction. Charge your food for 10 minutes before eating with these crystals nearby!

Prosperity:

Carry a blend of turquoise and ammonite to improve the prosperity energies around you for seven days.

Completeness:

Place the Eilat Stone over your sunlight-based plexus chakra when setting down to adjust your heart, brain, and body to feel great once more.

Determination:

Tiger's Eye is a great tool for encouraging self-control! For best results, make sure to wear this around the wrist of your dominant hand.

Workplace:

Place an amethyst group in your workplace to keep the energies liquid, clean, and positive for all who enter this space.

Troubling ISSUES:

When under stress, hold your Lepidolite in your dominant hand and focus on the favorable outcomes and perspectives!

WOUNDS:

Set carnelian and celestite inside two crawls of the sore and turn them in clockwise and counterclockwise motions, alternating between the two, to help heal wounds. Make sure to purge altogether a short time later. On the off chance that's conceivable, spot them on each side of the injury and work the energy to and fro together!

Compulsive worker:

To limit how much time the compulsive worker spends there, prepare a tree agate, rose quartz, and amber diamond solution, charge for two hours, and gently fog the entire area once a week.

Writing:

Try wearing a sodalite bracelet around the wrist that you use most often to compose in order to increase your writing capacity. On the off chance that you have an office, place this on your deck or work region!

YIN-YANG BALANCE:

Carry or wear an Eilat Stone for seven days, or however long it takes to adjust yin and yang energies.

Did you enjoy the book?

Please leave a review for others to enjoy it too.

Your review is valuable for us, please follow the link

https://amzn.to/3ggSkYM

www.ingramcontent.com/pod-product-compliance
Lightning Source LLC
Chambersburg PA
CBHW060843220526
45466CB00003B/1224